R3 Diet

R3 Diet

Reverse, Retrain,
Rebuild Your Body & Mind

Joy Brown

Edited by Julie Clay

Edited by Julie Clay
Cover Photography by Peggy Farren
Cover Design by Sarge Brown

Library of Congress Control Number: 2011904527
ISBN: Hardcover   978-1-4568-9095-7
               Softcover   978-1-4568-9094-0
               Ebook   978-1-4568-9096-4

This book was printed in the United States of America.

To order additional copies of this book, contact:
Xlibris Corporation
1-888-795-4274
www.Xlibris.com
Orders@Xlibris.com
96427

CONTENTS

Chapter 1   R U Ready for the truth? 15
Chapter 2   R U Ready for the R3 Diet?............................... 29
Chapter 3   R U Ready for the breakdown? 41
Chapter 4   R U Ready for power-packed fuel?.................. 63
Chapter 5   R U thirsty? 74
Chapter 6   R U Ready for the dangers?............................ 82
Chapter 7   R U Ready for the cleansers? 91
Chapter 8   R U Ready to get down & dirty?.................... 101
Chapter 9   R U Ready to change your mind?.................. 107
Chapter 10 R U Ready to grocery shop & store? 119
Chapter 11 R U Ready to hear from others?.................... 129
Chapter 12 R U listening to your body?........................... 139
Chapter 13 R U STILL listening to your body?................. 148
Chapter 14 R U ready to eat? 177

DISCLAIMER

DISCLAIMERS OF WARRANTY AND LIMITATION OF LIABILITY

This is provided by *R3 Diet* on an "as is" and "as available" basis. *R3 Diet* Book makes no representations or warranties of any kind, express or implied or the information, content, materials, or products mentioned. You expressly agree that your use of this information is at your sole risk. To the full extent permissible by applicable law, *R3 Diet* Book disclaims all warranties, express of implied, including, but not limited to, implied warranties or merchantability and fitness for a particular purpose. Anyone who is willing to try any suggestions from this book for health, fitness, nutrition, injury prevention, or anything relating to any of these areas, is responsible for doing their own due diligence before undertaking any new activity, or continuing a current activity relating to health, fitness, nutrition, injury prevention, or anything else in order to minimize the possibility of injury or death. The information shared herein has not been approved by the FDA, AMA nor any other health or regulatory agency. And therefore, anyone considering to use any of the information shared in this book should always consult a physician and/or a personal, certified fitness instructor before implementing any exercise routine or program—especially when significantly modifying one's physical fitness regime or lifestyle in any way.

BOOK DISCLAIMER

The ideas, concepts and opinions expressed in *R3 Diet* are intended to be used for educational purposes only. This book is sold with the understanding that author and publisher are not rendering medical advice of any kind, nor is this book intended to replace medical advice, nor to diagnose, prescribe or treat any disease, condition, illness or injury.

It is imperative that before beginning any diet or exercise program, including any aspect of the *R3 Diet*, you receive full medical clearance from a licensed physician.

Author and publisher claim no responsibility to any person or entity for any liability, loss, or damage caused or alleged to be caused directly or indirectly as a result of the use, application or interpretation of the material in this book.

The Food and Drug Administration has not evaluated the statements contained in the book, *R3 Diet*.

HEALTH SUPPLEMENTS DISCLAIMER

All supplements mentioned were designed for people who wish to supplement their normal diets with a wide variety of additional nutrients, some in amounts significantly higher than would be found in an ordinary diet. Your decision to supplement your diet with any nutritional supplements should be based on your own research and investigation or in consultation with your personal health care provider.

Ultimately, you must draw your own conclusion as to the efficacy of any nutrient. Any supplements mentioned in the *R3 Diet* book are not intended to diagnose, treat, prevent, mitigate or cure any diseases. If you are pregnant, nursing or have a known medical condition, are under a physician's care or taking prescription medications, we suggest consulting with your health care provider before starting on any high-potency supplementation program.

The Food and Drug Administration has not evaluated these statements.

ACKNOWLEDGEMENT

I would like to start by thanking God almighty, who created me with a specific purpose, gift and vision. I believe that the *R3 Diet* was birthed in me by God to change my health & life and the health and life of all who read and implement it around the world. Next I would like to thank my husband Sarge who has always supported my endeavors, but who supported me in the most magnificent & loving ways during this project. He encouraged me and even watched the kids & cleaned the house for me during some of my book revisions, all the while running and growing our health and fitness business. My husband is a talented risk taker that would do anything for his family and has an amazing quiet strength. I cannot thank him enough, and will always be grateful to have the most extraordinary husband a girl could dream of, who thoroughly completes me. I would like to thank my children, Destiny, Sevin , Loren & my step-daughter Tyler for their love and understanding. I know that you learn from people young and old in life and I have definitely learned a great deal from them. I am so glad that they are all different: Destiny has a big heart and smile and wants everyone to be happy. Sevin is charming and lives life with an enormous amount of passion. Loren is independent & quick-witted. Tyler is focused and determined. I love my family more than they will ever know! I would like to thank my mom, Diane for planting seeds of love, dreams, hope, perseverance, resilience, health and fitness in me and watering the seeds since childhood. I am thankful that I was able to see her attempt her goals and feel as if she passed the torch to me so that I could continue the race. My mom is strong, fierce and a fire cracker like none other! I would like to thank my editor Julie for all of her time and effort that she put into this project. She is also a working married mom with children and she devoted herself wholeheartedly to the *R3 Diet* book. Last but not least I would like to thank all my family, friends, clients and social network followers. If you have ever spoken or written a word to me, then you had an impact on my life. I value your input and thank you and expect great testimonials from you and all who read this book!

INTRODUCTION

I grew up with a mom who was passionate about health and fitness. I reluctantly let her dress me in leotards and leg-warmers as I even more reluctantly would do exercise routines with her for schools or organizations. Our house was filled with many health and fitness magazines, videos and books. I even remember her excitement during the grand opening of her fitness studio called, "De's Body Design". Although my mom planted a seed for that industry within me, I clearly did not recognize or accept it until years later.

After high school I wanted to study something that would define me and not my mom, so I went to school and became a Medical Assistant. I started off assisting a Gastroenterologist and then a Cardiologist. During that time I enrolled in college with a major in nursing. I quickly changed my field to Business Administration because I felt strongly about owning my own business, but was not sure in what field. During my school years and after earning my Bachelor's degree in Business Administration, I opened and quickly closed at least a dozen small businesses. It was difficult on my family, especially my husband who lost time and money in those ventures. I would laugh and tell him he "created a monster", because he was the one who told me I could do anything I wanted to do as long as I was passionate about it and gave it my all. Feeling discouraged about my last failed venture, I went into a state of depression for almost a year. I would get up, get my husband and kids off to work and school, and then crawl back in bed until they came home and I had to cook dinner. I really struggled with understanding my purpose here on earth. I often went to church and prayed for clarity and guidance. My life changed one night when I had a very vivid dream about working out with people outdoors.

I awoke to feeling of excitement and passion like I had never felt before! I told my husband about this dream, and we immediately starting researching how I could get trained and start a fitness business. Given my background working for a large gym, I knew that I wanted to create a different experience altogether. I went to California to get the necessary training and soon after my husband, who was an army sergeant, was called to active duty in the war on Iraq. He would be there for 18 months, so I had to start and grow our fledgling fitness company by myself. It was difficult, but I was finally doing something that made me feel ALIVE! However, the more I worked out with my clients, held conference calls and seminars, the more I noticed that there was one component of a healthy lifestyle that many were struggling with, and that was food.

I started having my clients journal their meals and turn them in for me to grade. I noticed that there were some common problems that plagued everyone, from stay-at-home moms to attorneys, and everything in between. These food issues were causing them mental grief, confusion, health issues and unfulfilled body weight goals. My initial reaction was to try already existing diet plans. I would study a plan and then we all would try it, journal it and I would study the results.

I started studying, testing and eliminating diet after diet. (The South Beach Diet, The Zone, The Bread of Life Diet, The Raw Food Vegan Diet, Eat Right 4 Your Type & The 5 Factor Diet, just to name a few.) I kept finding many holes in their execution and menus. Some diets compromised long term health for short term results (Atkins diet, anyone?), while others had high failure rates. Several diets were built as great dietary choices, but were nothing more than dietary disasters. After experimenting with 20 different diets, I knew there had to be a better way to design the optimal diet/fitness plan.

In the process I learned some AMAZING things about food and nutrition. I became a Certified Fitness Nutrition Coach, and aimed even higher. I was determined to if not find, then create the healthiest, body-sculpting eating plan that ever existed. *R3 Diet* is this goal fulfilled, and represents years of comparison, study, and ultimately, eating success. As I saw my clients constantly struggle with their eating habits. I knew I would be doing them an injustice by not sharing this important fact:

In order to reach one's health and fitness goals, food is 80% of the equation, while exercise is 20%.

CHAPTER 1

R U Ready for the truth?

Before considering how to solve a problem, it is important to make sure that the problem really exists. The following 2007 study shows the magnitude of the diet problem at hand: A team at Johns Hopkins University in Baltimore examined 20 studies published in journals and looked at national surveys of weight and behavior for their analysis, published in the Journal Epidemiologic Reviews. "Obesity is a public health crisis. If the rate of obesity and overweight continues at this pace, (then) by 2015, 75 percent of adults and nearly 24 percent of U.S. children and adolescents will be overweight or obese, and 86 percent of Americans could be overweight or obese by the year 2030," said Dr. Youfa Wang, who led the study. They defined adult overweight and obesity using a standard medical definition called body mass index. People with a BMI of 25 or above are considered overweight, while those with BMIs of 30 or above are obese and at serious risk of heart disease, diabetes and some cancers. Studies show that 66 percent of U.S. adults were overweight or obese in 2003 and 2004. May Beydoun, one of the researchers involved in the Johns Hopkins study, stated, "Obesity is likely to continue to increase, and if nothing is done, it will soon become the leading preventable cause of death in the United States."

Thanks to the average Western diet, known commonly as the Standard American Diet (aka ironically S.A.D.), people are trading the chance to be fit and healthy for a lifetime of sickness and disease. A skyrocketing amount of animal fats, unhealthy fats, and processed food has replaced fruit, fiber and plant-based foods in the SAD diet. Obesity rates have doubled in adults and tripled in children and adolescents over the last two decades, and diabetes, obesity's "Twin Epidemic" is devouring many of the same recipients. In order to get new results, we have to take new actions with a new mindset.

Three main reasons people frequently desire unhealthy foods:

1. **The Brain Reward System**—Food is a primary reward. High-calorie, highly palatable foods are typically found as being highly rewarding. Especially tasty foods elicit brain responses similar to those elicited by drugs of abuse such as cocaine and nicotine, pointing to a general involvement of the brain's "reward" system.
2. **Triggers**—A trigger is a prompting to eat something that serves no nutritional benefit to the body. There are trigger foods that entice you, either when you see them or hear of them. There are trigger times that seem to be common for the cravings. There are trigger places where you consume them. There are trigger thoughts/emotions that come up that make you automatically reach for the trigger foods.
3. **Addiction**—My personal definition of addiction is something that you do frequently, and although it is not in your best interest you can't seem to stop. Each time you put these unhealthy foods in your mouth, your taste buds grow used to them and your body prompts you to keep eating because it knows that digestion is occurring, yet **not finding nutrients**. That is why it is easy to polish off a whole bag of chips or cookies. The whole cycle will start over again each time you think of or encounter the undesirable food.

Reverse. Retrain. Rebuild . . . Consider the following questions:
Are you tired of seeing excess weight on your body?

Do you wonder if it's best to accept your current body since you can't reach your desired body?

Do you think that skinny people are just lucky and were born that way?

Are you sick of starting and failing diets? Do you feel hopeless in your efforts to eat properly?

Does your refrigerator and pantry look identical to your parents'?

Are most of your groceries pre-packaged bags and boxes?

Do you think that living a healthy lifestyle will constantly be an ongoing struggle filled with never-ending hunger pains?

Do you think that it costs more to eat healthy?

Do you want to quit dreaming of a healthy lifestyle and actually have one?

Well I have very good news for you! You now have in your hands **a powerful solution** to the above concerns! By applying the principles in this book, you will feel and look *amazing*, with extraordinary results in the fastest and safest way possible.

4-Pillars

My 4 pillars for success are 1.Food 2.Fitness 3.Supplements 4. Mindset (I want you to view these 4 pillars by this easy 4-piece puzzle analogy)

1. **Food** is the biggest piece of the puzzle.
2. **Fitness** is the actual act of putting the puzzle together.
3. **Supplements** are the glue that fills in the cracks of the puzzle.
4. **Mindset** is what is needed to complete the puzzle.

R3 Diet components:

Reverse Psychology & Sickness
Retrain Mind & Taste buds
Rebuild Body & Cells

Reverse psychology and how it helps you stick to the R3 eating plan

Reverse psychology is a persuasion technique involving the advocacy of a belief or behavior that is opposite to the one desired, with the expectation that this approach will encourage the subject of the persuasion to do what is desired: the opposite of what is suggested. This technique relies on the psychological phenomenon of reactance, in which a person has a negative emotional response in reaction to being persuaded, and thus chooses the option which is being advocated against.

This is very important in the eating plan because people generally know what "bad" foods are and know to best avoid them. However, the thought of completely eliminating these foods from their diet makes the average person *want them even more*. When they consume these foods they feel like a failure, which thwarts all efforts and motivation toward a healthy lifestyle. What follows is a lack of motivation and depression over losing control, then the fear of not knowing when or how bad the damage will be next time. They start to wonder why their willpower is not sufficient enough. (Note: Willpower is an intensely powerful yet temporary boost. You can use it in the beginning of your new healthy lifestyle strategy to get momentum going, but once it starts to subside you want to be able to depend on the new habits that have formed as a result of your new actions.)

The following is the reverse psychology strategy that the R3 Diet uses to demolish this problem:

The R3 Diet offers "Anything" foods for select days/times. Subconsciously you will not crave them nearly as much. If you do indulge with less than desirable foods at those times it will not be as enjoyable or as proportionately large because of the retraining and rebuilding that occurs when you are on the core routine meals. Yes, it is possible to completely retrain your taste buds to not even desire the bad stuff!

Reverse Sickness with Core Routine Meals:

Origin of sickness: We all live in a toxic environment. No matter where we live or how careful we are, we can't avoid environmental toxins. They are in the air we breathe, the food we eat and the water we drink all over the planet. High levels of pesticides & chemicals in processed foods are of particular concern. Free radicals are produced when our cells create energy and when we are exposed to pollutants or toxins such as cigarette smoke, alcohol or pesticides. If allowed to go unquenched, free radicals can cause damage to the body's cells. The cells that line the arteries, the fat cells in the blood, the immune cells and so on can all be affected by free radicals. And because of this, free radical damage (or oxidation) has been linked to the formation of every degenerative disease known including cancer, cardiovascular disease, cataracts and the aging process itself.

Free radicals are unstable chemicals formed in the body during normal metabolism or exposure to environmental toxins such as air, food and water pollution. Free radicals help our bodies to generate energy and fight infections, but when we have too many free radicals they attack healthy cells causing them to age prematurely. The action of rust is probably the best analogy of how excess free radicals work in our body.

Molecules called antioxidants can interact and stabilize free radicals, by donating their electrons to unpaired atoms, molecules, or ions. Moreover, antioxidants are able to donate their electrons to damaged DNA or fatty acids, and literally reverse the damage.

Some antioxidants, such as superoxide dismutase, catalase and gluthathione peroxidase, are synthesized by the body. They are actually antioxidant enzymes and a self-defense against free radicals.

The other antioxidants are obtained from food sources like vitamins (such as vitamins C and E), some minerals (such as selenium), and flavonoids, which are found in plants. Various fruits and vegetables are the best sources of antioxidants and flavonoids.

Benefits: The core routine meals are the raw, healthy, cleansing, nutrient-rich, energy igniting, anti-aging enhancing, beauty and weight-loss promoting/maintaining foods that will make up the bulk of your diet. Simply put, they are fruits and vegetables. These foods are designed to nourish you and keep you satiated throughout the day. They are full of phytonutrients, vitamins, minerals, antioxidants, amino acids and enzymes with which to enhance and maintain a healthy body. These meals will reset your "appetite thermostat" so you won't feel as hungry, thereby making it easier to stick with your eating plan. Also when it is time for you to eat your "anything meals", your body will naturally limit or quite possibly even *reject* the unsuitable foods.

Retrain taste buds:

You will be retraining your taste buds to appreciate and even crave the nourishing foods because of the consistency of the core routine meals. Remember: **What you give your body the most it also craves.** Taste buds are small receptors on your tongue that register what you've tasted, then relay the message to your brain. Most of the "buds" sit on the front raised part of your tongue but "buds" are divided into multiple sections.

The least of your taste sensation can be found towards the flatter back area of the tongue. These stations help to identify the five primary "tastes," which are sweet, sour, bitter, salty, and savory.

The great thing about taste buds is that we can change them, thus changing our entire eating habits, in as little as two to four weeks! This is why some diet programs utilize a detox system—to help steer you into a better eating direction with actual taste sensations.

Retrain mind:

For years you have trained your mind on your common eating habits. You probably walk through the grocery store being led by your subconscious on what to get, how to make it and how much to eat. Over 90 percent of your mental activity is subconscious. Also, Over 90 percent of them were installed during your early childhood by your primary caregivers. As a young child, you didn't have the psychological development to question what was true and what wasn't true so the most dominant thoughts and beliefs implicitly or explicitly expressed by your parents, guardians, teachers, respected elders and even society, were programmed onto your subconscious. You will now be consciously retraining your mind to encompass the habits of your new healthy agenda. You will also be provided with vital nutrients upon which our mental and emotional health depends.

Rebuild cells:

There are three major types of cells in blood—red blood cells (RBCs), white blood cells (WBCs) and platelets. Blood is a transportation of dissolved gases (carbon dioxide and oxygen), nutrients, enzymes, blood cells (WBCs 'leucocytes' and RBCs 'erythrocytes'), hormones and metabolic wastes.; Maintains and controls a normal PH and body temp of the body; Blood contains different types of white blood cells where each have specific roles in which they fight infections, toxins or remove cell debris. Platelets, also called thrombocytes, help in clotting of blood. They are essential in maintaining wear and tear of the body. The core routine meals will now give your blood cells a chance to rebuild and work more efficiently.

Rebuild body:

Our bodies are AMAZING! As soon as you start giving it what it wants, it rewards you by giving you what you want: A nicely toned body, unprecedented energy, youthful appearance, optimal health and much, much more!

Benefits of A Mainly Plant Based Diet

If you go to any hospital in the U.S. and ask the patients about their common eating routines, you will quickly notice that their diets typically include a much higher amount of meat and dairy foods to plant foods. Plant-based foods in their original, un-heated (uncooked) state are considered raw and alive. They are as much as 200-300% more nutritionally dense. These live foods (living foods) contain a wide range of vital life force nutrients (ie. vitamins, minerals, amino acids, oxygen) and live enzymes. Their nutritional properties are essential to the proper maintenance of human bodily functions and optimum health. Fruit is one of the healthiest natural foods in existence. It's very easy for the body to process and absorb the vitamins and minerals found in fresh fruit. A major benefit of vegetables is that they are low-calorie foods. Fruit and vegetables not only add a healthy dose of necessary nutrition and phytonutrients to the daily diet, they also contain antioxidants important for health and disease prevention. They add color as well. The compounds that give fruits and vegetables their color have unique nutritional properties, so by eating a wide array of colors, you can maximize these benefits, which in turn help your body to become and stay healthy. Fruits and vegetables are also great sources of fiber.

Research has proven that sufficient fiber in the diet offers a great many health benefits including aiding in digestion, lowering levels of cholesterol in the blood, reducing the risk of heart disease and stroke, and reducing the chances of some forms of cancer. In addition, fiber is thought to play an important role in controlling levels of blood sugar in diabetics. Fiber also helps dieters feel full while limiting the number of calories you consume. By eating more fruits and vegetables and fewer high-calorie foods, you'll find it much easier to control your weight and get all of your essential amino acids.

Our bodies require 20 different amino acids, eight of which we cannot produce ourselves. They are called the "essential" amino-acids because we need to obtain them through proper consumption of necessary foods. This is easy to do, as several different fruits and vegetables such as asparagus, broccoli, cauliflower, peas, celery, tomatoes, cantaloupe, strawberries, bananas, avocados and all green leafy vegetables each contain all of the eight essential amino acids, which are found in the plant proteins. Yes, plants have protein! Scientific studies have shown that plant-based proteins are also high in quality. These proteins are easier for the human body to assimilate and plant foods do not have many of the negative health implications associated with a diet rich in animal protein such as high cholesterol, high blood pressure and cardiovascular disease.

The very 1st pillar of my 4-pillar system is food. The right foods are fuel. This book is about using food in a way that propels us through life in a child-like, youthful, energetic and healthful way. You have eaten your way for "fill in the blank" years and now let's discuss step 1 of my "my way"!

30-Day Raw Foods Detox

Eating is 80% of the equation as it relates to reaching your health and fitness goals. With this in mind the 30-day raw foods detox is a very important 1st step before starting the R3 Diet. You have spent many years eating the Standard American Diet, causing the body to be full of toxins, and now you need a clean slate. The top four benefits of this detox are:

1. Flooding your system with lots of nourishing vitamin-and mineral-rich fruits and vegetables while pushing out all of the toxins
2. Retraining your taste buds to appreciate and desire healthy foods
3. Catapulting you out of fat-storing mode and into fat-burning mode.
4. Creating discipline to follow a healthy diet happily and easily

I have tested a one-, two- and three-week detox with my clients and there is something magical about the benefits of doing it for four weeks straight. It attests to the theory of needing 30 days to create a new habit. I have also noticed that those who do the detox before the diet tend to have an easier transition into the diet than those who don't.

30-Day Raw

This is the daily raw menu plan that you follow seven days/wk for the entire 30 days. If you are really up for a challenge, this is optimal and yields the greatest results.

Breakfast: Green Smoothie Meal
Lunch 1: Fruit Meal
Lunch 2: Veggie meal
Dinner: Veggie wrap/sandwich meal

Detox Meals

Breakfast: Green Smoothie Meal Blend 50% fruits and 50% vegetables and take between 30 minutes to two hours to drink. You want it to yield 20-60 ounces of green smoothie. Great vegetable sources are green leafy vegetables or celery and herbs. Great fruit choices include: bananas, strawberries, mango, peaches, blueberries, raspberries, blackberries, and pineapple. What's great is that the fruit list could go on and on. It is best to use fresh fruit; however you can mix in some frozen fruit periodically. Mix with some ice and one or two cups of water.

Lunch 1: A **fruit meal** should consist of no more than three different types of fruit at each meal. Fill up a dinner plate with fruit and eat. Remember: Raw meals should be served on dinner plates filled with nourishing fruits.

Lunch 2: A **veggie meal** will either be a salad (includes lettuce) or a veggie combo (excludes lettuce). It should include avocados one day and nuts/seeds the next (alternating between the two) (If you are allergic to nuts, exclude them). Drizzle with a healthy oil and vinegar or lemon juice, a healthy dressing or a fruit dressing like blended oranges and tomatoes. Remember: Raw meals should be served on dinner plates filled with plenty of nourishing vegetables.

Dinner: Veggie wrap/sandwich meal which is identical to the veggie meal, however you may add two pieces of Ezekiel, Genesis or Manna bread. These breads are made with sprouted grains and are not technically raw, but are baked at lower than normal temperatures.

Detox Rules

Absolutely NO sodas, coffee or alcohol on your detox days!

Absolutely NO snacking in between meals.

You may drink plenty of water and herbal teas throughout your detox. You should strive for an optimal 64 oz of water each day.

Eat fruit and/or veggie meals on dinner plates to ensure you are getting enough quantity.

Eat four times a day and know your exact eating times. For example: I eat my meals at 7:30a.m., 11a.m., 2:30p.m and 6p.m. By staying true to your times it helps a habit form and helps your metabolism run efficiently. Obviously it is okay if things happen where it is not exactly on point, but you do want it to be very close the majority of time. Fill in the blanks with your tentative four eating times:

Breakfast: 7:30 a.m. _____

Lunch 1: 11 a.m. _____

Lunch 2: 2:30 p.m. _____

Dinner: 6 p.m._____

Detox Symptoms

As the toxins exit your body, you will notice any or all of the following uncomfortable symptoms during the first week or more:

Headaches
Nausea
Constipation
Diarrhea
Flatulence
Light-headedness
Bad breath
Skin breakout
Irritability
Moodiness

Detox Rewards

By the third week of your detox, you should start noticing the following improvements:

Happiness
Increased energy
Mental alertness
Weight loss and/or inches lost
Sense of accomplishment
New appreciation of fruits and vegetables
Rejuvenation and reversed signs of aging
Improved memory
Enjoying a deep, sound sleep at night
Strengthened immune system
Natural bodily functions stabilized and normalized
Desire to exercise

Here are some of the frequent comments we have heard from our clients upon completion of the raw detox:

"I am craving more fruits & vegetables than I have in my entire life!"

"My triglycerides went from 187 to 86 in four weeks!"

"I can't believe I lost 15lbs and 20 inches in four weeks!"

"Our entire office did the challenge together and had such great results that we replaced the coffee maker with a blender. We are so much more productive, energetic and slim now!"

"At first I didn't think I could do the entire four weeks so I went to R3FitWorld.com for an accountability partner. I got more than enough support and finished the four weeks and surpassing my goals!"

"This detox helped me with ailments that I have been suffering from for years! I can't put into words how happy I am . . . I have my health back!"

"I started to notice improvements almost immediately!"

"I thought my diet was pretty decent and could not figure out why no matter what I did I couldn't lose weight. This was the jump start I needed. It seemed to melt off like butter!"

"This detox is the most powerful cleanse EVER! I wish I had known about it sooner!!!"

TOOLS (The following are highly recommended to R3-Arrange your kitchen)

Following the detox you are now ready to embark upon the *R3 Diet* for the ultimate body sculpting diet that brings unparalleled health and nutrition.

Success Tools for 30-Day Raw Detox and *R3 Diet*

Blender (Vitamix or Blendtec are excellent brands)
Knife set and cutting board
Juice Jar, thermos or air tight container for juices and/or smoothies
Cooler Tote Bag (to chill, carry and store your produce throughout the day)
R3 Eating Plan/Journal
Bragg's Vinaigrette
Ezekiel Bread/Wraps (2/day)
24-32 oz water bottle
Unsweetened herbal teas
Print resource-*R3 Diet* Book
Online resource-R3FitWorld.com

After the 1st 30 days you may also like to purchase

Juicer
Food processor (For slicing, grating, and shredding, especially large amounts, a food processor is your best friend.)
Dehydrator
Mandoline Plus (useful for rapidly producing multitudes of thin slices and julienne strips.)
Spiralizer (allows you to create spaghetti and spiral shapes from vegetables and fruit.)
Rice Cooker (For quickly cooking rice, beans & whole-grains)
Mason Jars (For soaking nuts or sprouting)

CHAPTER 2

R U Ready for the R3 Diet?

R3 Diet

Monday-Thursday

Breakfast: Juice or Green Smoothie

Lunch 1:   Green Smoothie or Fruit Meal

Lunch 2:   Fruit Meal or Salad w/nuts, avocado or small carb

Dinner: Cooked Meal: Carb meal or Protein meal w/cooked veggies
(Alternate one night carb, next night protein, etc.)

Friday-Sunday

Breakfast: Juice or Green Smoothie

Lunch 1:   Fruit Smoothie or Fruit Meal

Lunch 2:   Fruit Meal or Salad w/handful of nuts, avocado or carb

Dinner: Anything meal

Tips:

Juice: 15-30oz (Must be extracted from a juicer)

Smoothies: 20-60oz

Salads: Great carb options: Whole-grain bread, beans or sweet
potato. (Your hand is the serving size for the carb)

Plates: Consume raw meals on dinner plates and cooked meals on salad plates.

Dinner: It is always acceptable to have a salad with your dinner.

Anything meals: My personal "anything meal" usually consists of mixing a carb and protein item (ie. brown rice and scallops). The bottom line however is that you can eat whatever you choose for this meal.

Breakfast Fri-Sun: It is acceptable to substitute your juice/smoothie for a cooked, healthy breakfast periodically (ie. Whole grain pancakes, oatmeal or an omelet). *Note: Always have a minimum of two R3 meals on the weekend.

Desserts/Snacks: You can only have desserts/snacks on birthdays, holidays or special occasions, never to exceed 3x/Month! (The only exception is if one or more of the desserts is a raw dessert, you may consume a maximum of 4x/Month)

Guidelines for R3

This is considered a predominantly plant-based diet or a "high raw" diet. "High raw" means that most of the diet consists of raw foods. Raw foods are fresh and will be eaten simply. However it is also OK to eat "gourmet raw" foods that are vegetables, fruits, nuts, seeds and sprouted grains that are dehydrated and creatively prepared using no more than 116 degrees of heat. The natural enzymes remain alive thereby allowing easy digestion and encouraging deep detoxification and natural healing. I encourage simplicity by focusing mainly on fresh vegetables, fruit and nuts/seeds. However, it is acceptable to add dehydrated or gourmet raw to the eating plan a few times/wk.

Breakfast: Juice 15-30 ounces of fresh vegetables and apples and drink within 30 minutes or less. Great vegetable sources include carrots, cucumbers, celery, cabbage, green leafy vegetables and zucchini. Great add—ins would be beets, herbs, ginger, lemon and lime.

*   If you do not have a juicer, make blended salads as a substitute until you get a juicer. A blended salad is a mixture of raw, leafy greens and other foods blended together to make a smooth, creamy salad with a baby-food-like consistency making it pre-digested. Eating a salad prepared in this manner is quick and convenient, and increases absorption of important nutrients. You just toss some veggies into your blender and add maybe some herbs, an orange or a few dates. You can also go to some health food stores to have your produce freshly juiced on the spot, but obviously with time it will be more cost-effective & efficient for you to purchase your own juicer.

Lunch 1: **Green Smoothie Meal:** Blend 50% fruits and 50% vegetables and take between 30 minutes to 2 hours to drink. You want it to yield 20-60 ounces of green smoothie. Great vegetable sources are green leafy vegetables or celery and herbs. Great fruit choices include: bananas, strawberries, mangoes, peaches, blueberries, raspberries, blackberries, and pineapples. What's great is that the fruit list could go on and on. It is best to use fresh fruit; however you can mix in some frozen fruit periodically. Mix with some ice and one or two cups of water.

Lunch 2: **Fruit meals** should consist of no more than three different types of fruit at each meal. Fill up a dinner plate with fruit and eat.

Dinner: C (Carb) or P (Protein) Meals will be alternated each night. If you have whole-grain rice and steamed vegetables on Monday, you could have baked fish and steamed vegetables on Tuesday and so on.

Anything meals: There are no rules or guidelines for the "anything" meals, however review the proper food combining section and the seven-day sample section to know what is optimal.

- Eat four times a day and know your exact eating times.
- No more than one handful of nuts per day
- No more than three—five avocados per week
- Men will eat all meals on dinner plates. Women should eat raw meals on dinner plates and cooked meals on salad plates.

- **NEVER** compromise or change anything on the Monday –Thursday meals. , **This is a huge component of the retrain and rebuild** aspect of this diet, and is the key to the mastery of eating discipline, healthy fare appreciation and the abandonment of the bad cravings and binges.

Food Combining

The concept of proper food combining is a well-established, simple and practical approach to eating which provides many benefits. These include:

- Better digestion
- Increased energy
- Alertness
- Improved elimination
- Weight loss
- Sense of well being

If you eat the wrong combination of foods, your meal will not be digested completely, and therefore not provide the necessary nutrients to your cells. Instead, some of the foods will decompose in your stomach, potentially causing indigestion, dehydration, fatigue (because complicated combinations require much energy to digest), weight gain and other problems.

Basic Rules –

DO:

- Eat watery foods first (ie. juices before smoothies and smoothies before whole fruit)

- Eat proteins only with vegetables
- Eat starches/whole grains with vegetables and other starches/whole grains
- Eat fruit alone as a fruit meal, not between meals while other food is digesting in the stomach (may be added to green leafy vegetables and celery and sprouts)
- Eat melons alone

DO NOT:

- Eat protein foods and starches/whole grains together. Have them at separate meals.
- Eat fats and proteins together. Have them at separate meals.
- Drink beverages or even water during meals because it will dilute natural enzymes in your body.(avoid it a half an hour before through a half an hour after. You may take a few sips if needed during meal.)
- Mix dried sweet fruit, honey, maple syrup or bananas with nuts or seeds
- Mix sweet fruits with acid fruits. Here is a list of fruit categories:

Acid fruits: Blackberry, Grapefruit, Lemon/Lime, Orange, Pineapple, Plum (sour), Pomegranate, Raspberry, Sour Apple, Strawberry

Sub-Acid Fruit: Apple, Apricot, Blueberry, Cherry, Kiwi, Mango, Papaya, Peach, Pear, Plum (sweet), gooseberries

Sweet Fruit: Bananas, Dates, Currents, Figs, Fruit dried, Grapes, Papaya, Persimmons, Prunes, Raisins

Melon: Cantaloupe, Honey Dew, Papaya, Persian Melon, Musk Melon, Watermelon

Dried Fruits: Dried sweet fruits should be used sparingly. Use but one kind at a meal in small amounts. They should be combined only with sweet fruit and/or lettuce and/or celery.

Beans: Beans are high in carbohydrates, fairly rich in protein, and low in fat—or in other words, absolutely perfect for individuals who want to ingest high-performance food. The fiber in beans may also reduce appetite and assist people who are trying to lose weight. Beans also bring good supplies of calcium, copper, iron, zinc, phosphorus, potassium and magnesium into a health conscious person's body. However the following methods of preparing beans will help dramatically reduce flatulence and indigestion which is oftentimes associated with beans.

Bean Preparation Methods

Pre-soaking—Pre-soaking the beans and discarding the cooking water before final cooking, makes a big difference in digestibility. Here's how you do it.

Cover with water, at least 3 to 1 water to beans, since they swell up. Then let the beans sit at room temperature, at least 8 hours or overnight. If you are going to soak them for a full day you can change the soaking water halfway through.

Allow for dry beans expanding when soaked and cooked. One cup dried beans will yield 2 1/2 to 3 cups cooked beans, so be sure to allow for that. If you pre-soak, the swelling will take place while soaking, so you will know the finished volume when you cook. If you plan on cooking the beans from dry without soaking, be sure to allow extra water, and extra room in the pot, for the expansion.

Quick soak—After cleaning, put beans in water and bring to a boil, and boil them for about five minutes, then let them sit for one hour or more. Whichever method of soaking you use, drain and discard the soaking water and rinse the beans thoroughly before adding fresh water and cooking.

Very thorough cooking—This is the single most important factor in making beans easily digestible. Beans should be cooked until they are soft all the way through, with no firmness or crunchiness. Firm and crunchy beans look good on a plate but are hard to digest.

Boiling hard before main cooking—Whether you pressure cook or slow cook beans, it is a good idea to bring them to a rolling boil without pressure for about 10 minutes before using your main cooking method. This seems to help with digestion and can dramatically shorten the cooking time, especially when using a slow cooker.

Tips:

Wait on salt and acidic ingredients—Both salt and acidic ingredients such as tomatoes interfere with the process of beans becoming tender, so hold off adding them to the beans until they are thoroughly cooked.

Digestive Spices—Herbs and spices are packed with vitamins, trace minerals, and natural pharmaceuticals which alter the chemistry of food. Good ones for beans and lentils are fennel, coriander, cumin, ginger, turmeric (for chick peas, and Indian dhals), paprika, asafetida, cayenne, black pepper, and salt. Herbs such as thyme, bay leaf, basil, rosemary, marjoram, oregano, and cinnamon stick are also good. Consult recipes for proportions. Or experiment, but go easy until you hit on agreeable combinations and amounts. They aid with digestion but do not dominate the flavor. Japanese and Far East Asian cooking uses a piece of kombu or kelp, which is a kind of seaweed, cooked in with beans. It seems to help make beans a bit softer, thickens their cooking liquid a bit, and also enhances their flavor.

Combinations and Proportions of Foods—

Beans go really well with different forms of grains—rice, pasta, and breads (beans and rice, beans and tortillas, and bean soup/stews with pasta make wonderful, protein-complete meals). They seem to work best together when the amount of grains equals or exceeds the amount of beans. Grains and beans are usually found together in traditional cuisines around the world.

Chewing and savoring—Both beans and grains are foods where a lot of the digestive process starts in the mouth. Chewing beans and grains thoroughly, or savoring bean or pea soup broth in the mouth before swallowing, greatly reduces gas and makes digesting them a lot smoother. It also brings out more of their flavor and makes eating them more enjoyable.

Canned beans—When you use beans from a can or jar, make very sure that the beans are thoroughly cooked, soft and not crunchy. Drain and rinse the beans before adding them to whatever dish you are making. This makes them easier to digest. It gives the dish you add them to a cleaner and fresher taste, and it also seems to lengthen the time the leftovers stay good tasting in the fridge. You can also use spices like ginger and turmeric to aid digestion.

Nuts—Nuts contain enzyme inhibitors, which is why it's so important to soak them first. By soaking nuts and seeds, you release these toxic enzyme inhibitors and increase the life and vitality contained within them. Gluten breaks down so digestion is much easier. Phytic acid, which inhibits the absorption of vital minerals, is reduced. Just soak them overnight at room temperature in a mason jar, rinse and refrigerate. (See Soaking Chart for details)

Additional notes:

Chew your food thoroughly and make sure to enjoy the process and pleasure of eating.

The best way to eat grains is sprouted. Sprouted grains become alive with enzymes and oxygen. They become a pre-digested food. Other seeds and legumes should be sprouted as well. Soak at least three hours or overnight. (See Soaking Chart for details)

R3 FAQ (or the questions I am asked the most by clients)

What if I have a business lunch, can I switch my lunch 1 with my lunch 2 or dinner meal? Yes

What if a special occasion or holiday is on a weekday? You can switch your Fri-Sun "anything" meal with that Mon-Thurs in that case. For example: If you eat a traditional Thanksgiving meal including dessert on a Thursday, treat the following Friday like one of your "normal" Mon-Thurs R3 weekdays.

Can I have oatmeal or something other than juice or smoothie for breakfast on the weekends? Yes, It is ok to sometimes substitute your juice or smoothie for oatmeal, omelet, whole-grain pancakes or any other "traditional breakfast" that you may prefer. My Golden Rule #1: NEVER compromise/substitute anything on the R3 Diet during M-Thurs & ALWAYS have at least 2 R3 meals each day Fri-Sun.

How do you get enough protein on the raw detox? Your body doesn't use whole proteins—it must break these down into amino acids. Plant proteins generally break down for assimilation more quickly than animal proteins and are often found already in the form of amino acids. The following small list of fruits and vegetables contain all the amino acids not produced by the body: carrots, bananas, brussels sprouts, cabbage, cauliflower, corn, cucumbers, eggplant, kale, okra, peas, potatoes, summer squash, sweet potatoes and tomatoes.

What are the best sources of calcium? The best sources for calcium are: raw sesame seeds, all raw nuts, kelp, dulse, all leafy greens, and concentrated fruits such as figs, dates and prunes. Most fruit contains ample calcium.

I am busy, will this eating plan take away too much time from me? If you don't think that this eating plan is simple, good luck finding an easier one! Most of your meals are just peel, cut and eat! After you commit to it for a few months, you will see that there is no comparison.

What is the difference between subcutaneous fat and visceral fat? Subcutaneous fat is the fat we most see lying under the skin. Too much fat can cause the skin to become tight or stretched, and result in dreaded cellulite or a dimpled look of the skin. Unlike subcutaneous fat that lies just under the skin and is noticeable, visceral fat lies in the abdominal cavity under the abdominal muscle. Visceral fat is more dangerous than subcutaneous fat because it often surrounds vital organs. The more visceral fat one has, the greater the chance of developing Type 2 diabetes and heart disease.

Which common health/fitness words drive me bananas?

1. Moderation: Moderation is a word people use to abuse the food substance that they want to continue abusing. They will say, "_____is ok in moderation", knowing that there is nothing moderate about them consuming_____ 3x/day.
2. Try: "I will try that diet." Sorry, chances are you won't. Try is a cushion that people put down to land when they fall, which they know will be in the near future.
3. Baby steps: Everyone wants super fast results, but wants to take baby steps to get there. It does not work that way. Baby results . . . baby progress . . . Period!

What is the best way to eat fruit? Fruits are best eaten fresh, ripe and raw.

Is a tomato a fruit or a vegetable? To really figure out if a tomato is a fruit or vegetable, you need to know what makes a fruit a fruit, and a vegetable a vegetable. The big question to ask is, DOES IT HAVE SEEDS? If the answer is yes, then technically, (botanically) you have a FRUIT. From a botanical perspective, tomatoes are fruits. However, the masses refer to it as a vegetable.

What if I have failed at every single diet in the past? Dust off and move on! We have all failed at things in our past. It just means that we know how not to do something and our focus should be to keep moving forward until we find the answer.

What if no one else in my household eats healthy? I find that when one person seriously commits to a healthy lifestyle, it is only a matter of time before the other family members start to eat healthy. Many times the key can be making it taste, look and smell delicious.

What are some fun ways I can help my kids become interested in healthy foods? Two ways:

1. Let them help you prepare some of the meals.
2. Chopping their fruit and vegetables in different sizes or shapes makes them very appealing to kids.

Is it ok to skip meals on this plan? No, this is not a starvation diet. Obviously, if an urgent situation comes up every now and then that causes you to miss a meal it is ok. Just don't do it deliberately on a regular basis in an effort to lose more weight, because the opposite will usually happen.

What can I have if I get tired or hungry between meals? Have a glass of orange juice with a TBSP of brewer's yeast & wheat germ, blend & drink. The vitamin C of the citrus juice boosts the antioxidant factors in the brewer's yeast & wheat germ.

Can this way of eating get boring? You think that if you plan all of your meals around a meat based diet that means variety? It does not! You would still just choose between beef, chicken, pork, turkey or fish. There are thousands of different fruits and vegetables to choose from on a mainly plant-based diet.

What is the average time it should take to prepare the meals? It should take 30 minutes or less to prepare all of your meals, unless you are following some new complicated recipe(s).

What are your thoughts on whey or soy protein powders? I am not an advocate for whey or soy protein powders since many of them are highly processed and cause gas and bloating at the least.

What are the healthiest salts to use? Celtic sea salt and Himalayan sea salt

What are the healthiest natural sweeteners to use? Ripe fruit is the best way for us to satisfy a sweet tooth. However the following "sweeteners" can be used 3x/Month max: Jerusalem artichoke syrup, Yacon syrup, Organic Maple Syrup, Sucanat, date sugar, coconut sugar, raw honey, Agave nectar & fresh whole Stevia leaves, dried leaves or dried leaf powder (avoid white Stevia powder & liquid drops since they are highly processed).

Do you have to ALWAYS follow the food combining rules? No, use it as a guide to follow most of the time, but on a Saturday for instance if you want a smoothie with watermelon (which is best eaten alone) mixed with bananas and strawberries . . . go for it!

Does it cost more to eat healthy? No, obviously it saves you in the long run on medical expenses and prescribed drugs, but it also does not have to cost more now in your current lifestyle.

CHAPTER 3

R U Ready for the breakdown?

All the energy we need for life as well as for exercise comes from the food we eat and the *fluids* we drink. These nutrients are commonly broken into three classes:

- Carbohydrates
- Fats
- Proteins

Each category of food is important for health and we should all consume foods from each category. The ratios in which we need to consume these foods, however, are often the topic of a debate.

The Truth about Carbohydrates (60% of the calories in your diet should come from carbs)

Carbohydrates are the main source of energy and comprise the main bulk of the average human diet. For your brain, heart and nervous system to function properly, a constant supply of carbohydrates is needed. Once digestion has occurred, all forms of carbohydrates are converted into a sugar called glucose. Glucose is the main source of energy for muscles and other parts of the body.

Carbohydrates are divided into three groups:

- Monosaccharides: glucose, fructose, galactose (micro-molecular)
- Disaccharides: sucrose, lactose, maltose (micro-molecular)
- Polysaccharides: starch, glycogen, cellulose (macro-molecular)

The different types of carbohydrates found in foods are all transformed in the body to glucose. A high storage of carbohydrates in the form of glycogen helps keep you feeling energetic and ready for physical activities. Carbohydrates include starches, sugars, and dietary fiber. Starch and sugar supply the body with energy. Dietary fiber provides bulk to the diet, which stimulates regular elimination from the bowel. Carbohydrates are quickly converted to glucose which is alternatively referred to as the blood sugar. Glucose is used in two ways once it is absorbed into the blood stream. One, it is taken to the muscle sites for synthesis into energy. Secondly, it is further converted to glycogen, a chemical substance usually stored in the muscle cells and in the liver as an emergency measure against lack of energy in the body. Adequate carbohydrate intake also helps prevent protein from being used as energy. If the body doesn't have enough carbohydrates, then protein is broken down to make glucose for energy.

Because the primary role of protein is as the building blocks for muscles, bone, skin, hair, and other tissues, relying on protein for energy (by failing to take in adequate carbohydrates) can limit your ability to build and maintain tissues. Complex carbohydrate foods provide the chemical links necessary to burn off body fat. In fact, if your carbohydrate intake is too low, you cannot completely break down your body fat and it will actually store fat for reserve. This inability makes it difficult for you to shed extra pounds. It also means that you build up toxic wastes (ketone bodies) in your system, causing headaches, dehydration, and overwhelming hunger pangs.

The best sources of carbohydrates include whole grains, vegetables, fruits and beans/legumes. These are complex carbohydrates that also provide needed vitamins, minerals, fiber and a whole host of phytonutrients which have many health benefits. Carbohydrates that have been highly processed such as snack foods, bakery items and sodas provide calories but are low in fiber and many important nutrients. When you think of carbs, think of fiber as well. Our body requires sufficient amounts of fiber for maintenance of good health and smooth functioning of all the body parts. Fiber rich foods form a significant constituent of our diet and are beneficial to us in various ways. Fibers are nothing but the part of the plant that support the position of the plant. By dietary fibers, one means the cell wall parts of a plant. This includes hemicellulose, lignin, beta-glucans, cellulose, gums and fructans. Some of the richest sources of fibers are fruits, vegetables and grains.

Benefits of Fiber

- Fiber helps in relieving constipation, softening stools as they pass through the intestinal tract. This in turn, enables regular bowel movements.
- There are two types of fibers, soluble and insoluble. The soluble ones are beneficial for people suffering from diabetes. Such people usually absorb sugar in high amounts and this poses harm to their normal blood sugar levels. By taking soluble fibers, these amounts go down, thereby controlling the blood sugar levels in the body.
- Fiber aids in proper digestion of food and also relief from a variety of digestive disorders, such as irritable bowel syndrome and hemorrhoids.
- Fiber rich foods also aid in the weight loss, as a person usually takes a long time in chewing them and therefore, this contributes in the prevention of over eating. These foods also keep your stomach full for a long time and therefore you do not feel as hungry.
- Fiber helps to prevent cardiovascular diseases, cancer, gallstones, kidney stones, high blood pressure, rapid aging and high cholesterol levels.

- **Carbs and the brain:** Dr. Norberto Cysne Coimbra M.Sc., Ph.D., Laboratory of Neuroanatomy and Neuropsychobiology, says, "Your brain cells need two times more energy than the other cells in your body." Neurons, the cells that communicate with each other, have a high demand for energy because they're always in a state of metabolic activity. Even during sleep, neurons are still at work repairing and rebuilding their worn out structural components. They are manufacturing enzymes and neurotransmitters that must be transported out to the very ends of their nerve branches, some that can be several inches, or feet, away.
- Most demanding of a neuron's energy, however, are the bioelectric signals responsible for communication throughout the nervous system. This nerve transmission consumes one-half of all the brain's energy (nearly 10% of the whole body's energy). Most of us have discovered that thinking can be tiring, even exhausting. As the primary source of energy in the human brain, glucose can be rapidly used up during mental activity.
- Some interesting research has shown that mental concentration actually drains glucose from a key part of the brain associated with memory and learning—underscoring just how crucial this blood sugar is for proper brain function.

The Truth about Fat—30% of the calories in your diet should come from fat

The main purpose of fats in the body is to serve as a storage system and reserve supply of energy. During periods of low food consumption, fat reserves in the body can be mobilized and broken down to release energy. Fats serve as an insulation material to allow body heat to be conserved. They also line and protect delicate internal organs from physical damage. Fats in the diet can be converted to other lipids that serve as the main structural material in the membranes surrounding our cells. Fats are also used in the manufacture of some steroids and hormones that help regulate proper growth and maintenance of tissue in the body.

Unfortunately, some people mistakenly believe that consuming fat makes you fat. The food industry has capitalized on this belief by producing rows of grocery store shelves and freezers filled with low-fat, no-fat fake foods. Most low-fat, fat-free, 'diet' products, advertised as such, simply are not very good for us are nutritionally inferior to their less-processed, full-fat counterparts; something has to replace fat and usually it's sugar, corn syrup sweeteners, or chemicals.

The Truth about Meat Products
(Excerpt from *Eat Wild* by Jo Robinson)

Virtually all the meat, eggs, and dairy products that you find in the supermarket come from animals raised in confinement in large facilities called CAFOs or "Confined Animal Feeding Operations." These highly mechanized operations provide a year-round supply of food at a reasonable price. Although the food is cheap and convenient, there is growing recognition that factory farming creates a host of problems, including:

- Animal stress and abuse
- Air, land, and water pollution
- The unnecessary use of hormones, antibiotics, and other drugs
- Low-paid, stressful farm work
- The loss of small family farms
- Food with less nutritional value

Unnatural diets. Animals raised in factory farms are given diets designed to boost their productivity and lower costs. The main ingredients are genetically modified grain and soy that are kept at artificially low prices by government subsidies. To further cut costs, the feed may also contain "by-product feedstuff" such as municipal garbage, stale pastry, chicken feathers, and candy. Until 1997, U.S. cattle were also being fed meat that had been trimmed from other cattle, in effect turning herbivores into carnivores. This unnatural practice is believed to be the underlying cause of BSE or "mad cow disease."

Animal stress. A high-grain diet can cause physical problems for ruminants—cud-chewing animals such as cattle, dairy cows, goats, bison, and sheep. Ruminants are designed to eat fibrous grasses, plants, and shrubs—not starchy, low-fiber grain. When they are switched from pasture to grain, they can become afflicted with a number of disorders, including a common but painful condition called "subacute acidosis." Cattle with subacute acidosis kick at their bellies, go off their feed, and eat dirt. To prevent more serious and sometimes fatal reactions, the animals are given chemical additives along with a constant, low-level dose of antibiotics. Some of these antibiotics are the same ones used in human medicine. When medications are overused in the feedlots, bacteria become resistant to them. When people become infected with these new, disease-resistant bacteria, there are fewer medications available to treat them.

Caged pigs, chickens, ducks and geese. Most of the nation's chickens, turkeys, and pigs are also being raised in confinement. Typically, they suffer an even worse fate than the grazing animals. Tightly packed into cages, sheds, or pens, they cannot practice their normal behaviors, such as rooting, grazing, and roosting. Laying hens are crowded into cages that are so small that there is not enough room for all of the birds to sit down at one time. An added insult is that they cannot escape the stench of their own manure. Meat and eggs from these animals are lower in a number of key vitamins and omega-3 fatty acids.

Environmental degradation. When animals are raised in feedlots or cages, they deposit large amounts of manure in a small amount of space. The manure must be collected and transported away from the area, an expensive proposition. To cut costs, it is dumped as close to the feedlot as possible. As a result, the surrounding soil is overloaded with nutrients, which can cause ground and water pollution. When animals are raised outdoors on pasture, their manure is spread over a wide area of land, making it a welcome source of organic fertilizer, not a "waste management problem."

What is the healthiest choice? When you choose to eat meat, eggs, and dairy products from animals raised on pasture, you are improving the welfare of the animals, helping to put an end to environmental degradation, helping small-scale ranchers and farmers make a living from the land, helping to sustain rural communities, and giving your family the healthiest possible food. It's a win-win-win-win situation.

MEAT: Grass-fed and finished meats are lower in fat, contain a healthier balance of Omega-3 to Omega-6 fatty acids, plus they're higher in Conjugated Linoleic Acid (CLA), beta carotene, and vitamins A and E.

MILK: Pasteurization is a quick heat process designed to kill unpleasant bacteria and protect us against infectious diseases. The heat destroys amino acids, vitamins and minerals. Raw milk naturally contains good bacteria that help to digest the lactose in milk . . . when you pasteurize the milk you kill the good bacteria and then when you can't digest the milk you think you're lactose intolerant. Last but not least, pasteurization destroys all the enzymes in milk. On the other hand raw milk contains lactic-acid-producing bacteria that protect against pathogens. It contains milk's natural and full array of vitamins and minerals. It contains the enzymes your body uses to help digest it, easing your pancreatic load and preventing degenerative diseases. Best options: Organic, raw, whole, unpasteurized, unhomogenized, hormone and antibiotic free, grass-fed cow's milk or goat's milk.

BUTTER: Cream is the raw material for butter. Butter is a partially saturated fat, just like margarine. However, butter is a natural product that does not contain trans-fatty acids. Real butter has a positive health impact. Your best option is organic and raw butter.

There are many vitamins found in saturated animal fats which are integral to the strengthening of the immune system and the warding off of many diseases including cancer. Studies have shown that butter can have a positive effect on arthritis and can also lessen the risk of osteoporosis, and thyroid gland problems, and can promote good gastrointestinal health. Butter actually aids in the absorption of beta-carotene and other vitamin A related nutrients (plus vitamins D, E and K). Butter also contains the following:

- Conjugated Linoleic Acid (CLA)—helps your heart function better by utilizing fatty reserves for energy and reducing weight.
- Sphingolipids—assists in inhibiting cancer
- Stearic acid—lowers saturated fat
- Butyric acid—reduces chronic inflammatory conditions that help decrease the risk of colon cancer
- Myristic and lauric acid—raise your good cholesterol, aka HDL.

The same organic and grass fed guidelines above should apply to the following full fat dairy options: Cheese, eggs (omega 3 enriched), kefir, cottage cheese and yogurt (with active cultures). Resource: Local health food store or Organicpastures.com

COCONUT OIL

The following are quotes from Bruce Fife, N.D. on the power of coconut oil:

You have short-chain fatty acids (SCFA), medium-chain fatty acids (MCFA), and long-chain fatty acids (LCFA). Another term you will often see in reference to fatty acids is triglyceride. Three fatty acids joined together make a triglyceride, so you may have short-chain triglycerides (SCT), medium-chain triglycerides (MCT), or long-chain triglycerides (LCT).

The vast majority of the fats and oils you eat, whether they are saturated or unsaturated or come from an animal or a plant, are composed of long-chain triglycerides. Probably 98 to 100% of all the fats we eat consist of LCT. Coconut oil is unique because it is composed predominately of MCT. The size of the fatty acid is extremely important because physiological effects of medium-chain fatty acids in coconut oil are distinctly different from the long-chain fatty acids more commonly found in our diet. It's the MCT in coconut oil that make it different from all other fats and for the most part gives it its unique character and healing properties. Almost all of the medium-chain triglycerides used in research, medicine, and food products come from coconut oil. For at least five decades researchers have recognized that the MCT were digested differently than other fats. This difference has had important applications in the treatment of many digestive and metabolic health conditions and since that time MCT have been routinely used in hospital and baby formulas.

The digestive health advantages of MCT over LCT are due to the differences in the way our bodies metabolize these fats. Because the MCT molecules are smaller, they require less energy and fewer enzymes to break them down for digestion. They are digested and absorbed quickly and with minimal effort.

MCT are broken down almost immediately by enzymes in the saliva and gastric juices so that pancreatic fat-digesting enzymes are not even essential. Therefore, there is less strain on the pancreas and digestive system. This has important implications for patients who suffer from digestive and metabolic problems. Premature and ill infants especially whose digestive organs are underdeveloped, are able to absorb MCT with relative ease, while other fats pass through their systems pretty much undigested. People who suffer from malabsorption problems such as cystic fibrosis, and have difficulty digesting or absorbing fats and fat soluble vitamins, benefit greatly from MCT. They can also be of importance to people suffering from diabetes, obesity, gallbladder disease, pancreatitis, Crohn's disease, pancreatic insufficiency, and some forms of cancer.

As we get older our bodies don't function as well as they did in earlier years. The pancreas doesn't make as many digestive enzymes, our intestines don't absorb nutrients as well, the whole process of digestion and elimination moves at a lower rate of efficiency. As a result, older people often suffer from vitamin and mineral deficiencies. Because MCT are easy to digest and improve vitamin and mineral absorption they should be included in the meals of older people. This is easy to do if the meals are prepared with coconut oil.

In the digestive system MCT are broken down into individual fatty acids (MCFA). Unlike other fatty acids, MCFA are absorbed directly from the intestines into the portal vein and sent straight to the liver where they are, for the most part, burned as fuel much like a carbohydrate. In this respect they act more like carbohydrates than like fats.

Other fats require pancreatic enzymes to break them into smaller units. They are then absorbed into the intestinal wall and packaged into bundles of fat (lipid) and proteins called lipoproteins. These lipoproteins are carried by the lymphatic system, bypassing the liver, and then dumped into the bloodstream, where they are circulated throughout the body. As they circulate in the blood, their fatty components are distributed to all the tissues of the body. The lipoproteins get smaller and smaller, until there is little left of them. At this time they are picked up by the liver, broken apart, and used to produce energy or, if needed, repackaged into other lipoproteins and sent back into the bloodstream to be distributed throughout the body. Cholesterol, saturated fat, monounsaturated fat, and polyunsaturated fat are all packaged together into lipoproteins and carried throughout the body in this way. In contrast, medium-chain fatty acids are not packaged into lipoproteins but go to the liver where they are converted into energy. Ordinarily they are not stored to any significant degree as body fat. Medium-chain fatty acids produce energy. Other dietary fats produce body fat.

Because of the above advantages, coconut oil has been a lifesaver for many people, particularly the very young and the very old. It is used medicinally in special food preparations for those who suffer digestive disorders and have trouble digesting fats. For the same reason, it is also used in infant formula for the treatment of malnutrition. Since it is rapidly absorbed, it can deliver quick nourishment without putting excessive strain on the digestive and enzyme systems and help conserve the body's energy that would normally be expended in digesting other fats. Medium-chain triglycerides comprise a major ingredient in most infant formulas commonly used today.

Eating foods containing MCT is like putting high octane fuel into your car. The car runs smoother and gets better gas mileage. Likewise, with MCT your body performs better because it has more energy and greater endurance. Because MCFA are funneled directly to the liver and converted into energy, the body gets a boost of energy. And because MCFA are easily absorbed by the energy-producing organelles of the cells, metabolism increases. This burst of energy has a stimulating effect on the entire body.

The fact that MCT digest immediately to produce energy and stimulate metabolism has led athletes to use them as a means to enhance exercise performance. Studies indicate this may be true. In one study, for example, investigators tested the physical endurance of mice who were given MCT in their daily diet against those that weren't. The study extended over a six-week period. The mice were subjected to a swimming endurance test every other day. They were placed in a pool of water with a constant current. The total swimming time until exhaustion was measured. While at first there was little difference between the groups of mice, those fed MCT quickly began to out-perform the others and continued to improve throughout the testing period. Tests such as this demonstrated that MCT had the ability to enhance endurance and exercise performance, at least in mice.

In another study using humans, conditioned cyclists were used. The cyclists pedaled for three hours. During the last hour they were each given a beverage to drink. Those who received beverages containing MCT outperformed the others. Because of studies like these many of the sports drinks and energy bars sold at health food stores contain MCT to provide a quick source of energy.

It's easy to see why athletes would be interested in gaining greater endurance and energy, but what about non-athletes? MCT can do the same for them. If eaten regularly MCT can provide a boost in energy and performance of daily activities. Would you like to increase your energy level throughout the day? If you get tired in the middle of the day or feel you lack energy, adding coconut oil to your daily diet may provide you with a much needed boost to help carry you through.

Besides increasing your energy level, there are other very important benefits that results from boosting your metabolic rate: it helps protect you from illness and speeds healing. When metabolism is increased, cells function at a higher rate of efficiency. They heal injuries quicker, old and diseased cells are replaced faster, and young, new cells are generated at an increased rate to replace worn-out ones. Even the immune system functions better.

Several health problems such as obesity, heart disease, and osteoporosis are more prevalent in those people who have slow metabolism. Any health condition is made worse if the metabolic rate is slower than normal, because cells can't heal and repair themselves as quickly. Increasing metabolic rate, therefore, provides an increased degree of protection from both degenerative and infectious illnesses.

References:

1. Thampan, P.K. 1994. Facts and Fallacies About Coconut Oil. Asian and Pacific Coconut Community, p.8
2. Kiyasu G.Y., et al. 1952. The portal transport of absorbed fatty acids. Journal of Biological Chemistry 199:415
3. Fushiki, T. and Matsumoto, K. 1995, Swimming endurance capacity of mice is increased by chronic consumption of medium-chain triglycerides. Journal of Nutrition 125:531

The Truth about Protein—10% of the calories in your diet should come from protein.

Protein is essential to our bodies' normal functions. It assists in synthesizing enzymes and hormones, maintaining fluid balance, and regulating such vital functions as building antibodies against infection, blood clotting, and scar formation. Protein is also a building block for our muscles, bones, cartilage, skin, hair, and blood. Although very beneficial in the right amounts, most Americans already eat more protein than their bodies need. And eating too much protein can increase health risks.

DIETARY protein requirements have been a hotly contested issue throughout the brief history of modern nutritional science. Scientific evidence indicates adults require no more than 10-15% of their daily caloric intake from protein. But, popular diet books like *Enter the Zone, Protein Power* and *Dr. Atkins New Diet Revolution* persist in keeping the high-protein myth alive, recommending intake levels at 30% and higher.

Ron Brown, author of *The Body Fat Guide,* takes a completely different approach in determining protein requirements. He claims nature's answer to the question of how much protein we need lies within a woman's breast!

"Human breast milk contains approximately 10% of calories from protein," points out Brown. "This supplies all the protein needs during infancy, the time of a human's life when protein needs are the highest. On a diet of 10% protein, an infant will double its weight in six months and triple its weight in a year. How can an adult who is not building new tissue at the same rate possibly need a higher percentage of protein than this?" Brown says human milk, with less than one half the protein of cow's milk, contains the lowest percentage of calories from protein of all mammals. "The amount of protein in each species of mammal milk is matched to the normal growth rate of that species' offspring," says Brown. "Human infants grow much slower than calves."

Protein in 100 grams of Mammal Milk		
Mammal	Grams	% of Calories
Human	1.6	9.56
Cow	3.55	21.19
Dog	11.2	31.20
Swine	5.9	23.39
Sheep	6.5	24.14
Goat	4.3	22.84
Mare	1.3	13.40
Rabbit	15.5	37.69
Buffalo	4.4	17.55
Camel	3.6	24.04

Commenting on high-protein weight-loss diets, Brown says, "For weight-loss purposes, it's true that if you consume your usual maintenance amount of protein on a diet that is below your normal maintenance caloric intake level, this automatically increases the percentage of calories from protein in your diet. Yet, this still works out to a much lower percentage of calories from protein compared to the often recommended 30% or more on an unbalanced high-protein diet."

"For example, protein requirements are usually calculated at .8 grams per kilo of bodyweight. But, this amount of protein is twice the normal maintenance amount to cover cases where extra protein is required for growth purposes, such as pregnancy, lactation, etc. A 154-lb (70 kilograms) person on a well-balanced reduced-calorie diet of 1500 calories a day, who is not growing extra tissue and has no need for additional protein beyond maintenance purposes, requires only .4 grams of protein per kilo of bodyweight (28 grams). At 4 calories per gram of protein, this works out to 112 calories from protein or about 7% of overall calories from protein on a 1500-calorie diet." So why do popular diets stress high protein intake? Brown responds, "Because the body has a difficult time deriving energy from protein. Protein is designed to meet our growth, repair and reproductive needs, not our energy needs."

When you replace a normal balance of foods with protein, you cut back your overall energy intake. This makes it easier for people to lose weight. In addition, excess protein can cause a toxic response in your body which, like nicotine and caffeine, temporarily elevates your metabolism and burns more calories. Brown warns there is a high price to pay when relying on high-protein diets. In addition to contributing to liver and kidney problems, he cites a recent *National Institutes of Health* report which claims excess protein intake increases calcium excretion, causing osteoporosis. "And the weight comes back when you return to a normally balanced diet," adds Brown. "The temporary weight loss of an unbalanced high-protein diet is not a substitute for weight management skills and proper lifestyle habits."

Amino Acids=The Structural Units That Make Up Proteins

Amino Acids—L-Threonine, L-Valine, L-Methionine, L-Isoleucine, L-Leucine, L-Phenylalanine, L-Histidine, L-Lysine, L-Arginine, L-Aspartic acid, L-Serine, L-Glutamic acid, L-Proline, L-Glycine, L-Alanine, L-Tyrosine, L-Cysteine, L-5HTP

L-THREONINE—is required to help maintain the proper protein balance in the body, as well as assist in the formation of collagen and elastin in the skin.

L-VALINE—has a stimulating effect and is needed for muscle metabolism, repair and growth of tissue and maintaining the nitrogen balance in the body.

L-METHIONINE—assists in the breakdown of fats and thereby prevents the build-up of fat in the arteries, as well as assisting with the digestive system and removing heavy metals from the body since it can be converted to cysteine, which is a precursor to gluthione, which is of prime importance in detoxifying the liver.

L-ISOLEUCINE—promotes muscle recovery after physical exercise and on its own it is needed for the formation of hemoglobin as well as assisting with regulation of blood sugar levels as well as energy levels. It is also involved in blood-clot formation.

L-LEUCINE—helps with the regulation of blood-sugar levels, the growth and repair of muscle tissue (such as bones, skin and muscles), growth hormone production, wound healing as well as energy regulation. It can assist to prevent the breakdown of muscle proteins that sometimes occur after trauma or severe stress.

L-PHENYLALANINE—is used in elevating the mood since it is so closely involved with the nervous system, as well as help with memory and learning and has been used as an appetite suppressant.

L-HISTINDINE—is a precursor of histamine, and a compound released by immune system cells during an allergic reaction. It is needed for growth and for the repair of tissue, as well as the maintenance of the myelin sheaths that act as protector for nerve cells. It is further required for the manufacture of both red and white blood cells, and helps to protect the body from damage caused by radiation and in removing heavy metals from the body. In the stomach, histindine is also helpful in producing gastric juices, and people with a shortage of gastric juices or suffering from indigestion, may also benefit from this nutrient.

L-LYSINE—is required for growth and bone development in children, assists in calcium absorption and maintaining the correct nitrogen balance in the body and maintaining lean body mass. Furthermore it is needed to produce antibodies, hormones, enzymes, collagen formation as well as repair of tissue.

L-ARGININE—is extremely useful in enhancing the immune system, and it increases the size and activity of the thymus gland, which is responsible for manufacturing T lymphocytes—the much talked about T-cells, which assist the immune system. For this reason it might be an important nutrient for people suffering from AIDS and other malignant diseases which suppress the immune system.

L-ASPARTIC ACID—is required by the nervous system to maintain equilibrium and is also required for amino acid transformation from one form to the other which is achieved in the liver.

L-SERINE—is required for the metabolism of fat, tissue growth and the immune system as it assists in the production of immunoglobulins and antibodies.

L-GLUTAMIC ACID—is an important excitatory neurotransmitter, and glutamic acid is also important in the metabolism of sugars and fats. It can be used as fuel in the brain, and can attach itself to nitrogen atoms in the process of forming glutamine, and this action also detoxifies the body of ammonia. This action is the only way in which the brain can be detoxified from ammonia.

L-PROLINE—improves skin texture and aids collagen formation and helps contain the loss of collagen during aging. Collagen in the skin contains hydroxyproline and hydroxylysine, which is formed from proline and lysine, in which ascorbic acid seems to be important in this conversion. Collagen contains about 15 % proline. It is also thought to be important in the maintenance of muscles, joints and tendons.

L-GLYCINE—is required to build protein in the body and synthesis of nucleic acids, the construction of RNA as well as DNA, bile acids and other amino acids in the body. It is further found to be useful in aiding the absorption of calcium in the body.

L-ALANINE—is required for the metabolism of glucose and tryptophan, and beta-alanine is a constituent of vitamin B5 (pantothenic acid) as well as coenzyme A.

L-TYROSINE—the action of this amino acid in brain functions is clear with its link to dopamine as well as norepinephrine, but it is also helpful in suppressing the appetite and reducing body fat, production of skin and hair pigment, the proper functioning of the thyroid as well as the pituitary and adrenal gland. It is used for stress reduction and may be beneficial in narcolepsy, fatigue, anxiety, depression, allergies, headaches as well as drug withdrawal.

L-CYSTEINE—Your skin, as well as detoxification of your body, requires cysteine. It is found in beta-keratin, the main protein in nails, skin as well as hair. It not only is important in collagen production but also assists in skin elasticity and texture. Cysteine is also required in the manufacture of the amino acid taurine and is a component of the antioxidant gluthione. It is useful to detoxify the body from harmful toxins and help protect the brain and liver from damage from alcohol, drugs etc. It has also been found that it may help in strengthening the protective lining of the stomach as well as intestines, which in turn may help prevent damage caused by aspirin and similar drugs.

L-5HTP—converts into serotonin in the brain. Serotonin is an important brain chemical involved in mood, behavior, appetite, and sleep.

COUNTING CALORIES

In its most technical terms a calorie can be defined as a unit of measurement that is used to indicate the potential amount of energy provided to the body by a particular food. Also known as kilocalories (= 1000 calories), which the amount of energy that is needed to raise the temperature of 1 kilogram of water 1 degree Celsius. In its simplest form, a calorie can be considered just a unit of energy.

The whole idea of counting calories is only a few decades old. During the Cold War, a scientist began burning different types of food and measuring how much energy was released to try to set a baseline for which foods had how many calories. The scientist published his work and within a year or two, diet books began noting the caloric totals of different kinds of food and the obvious diet implications were obvious. Within ten years, calories were widely considered to be the basis for how you can control your weight down to the letter. It is incredible to think that this method of measuring is so new, but it wasn't that long ago that no one had any idea what a calorie even was.

When most Americans fail at dieting, it isn't because of lack of effort. A recent poll showed that while over two thirds of all Americans consider the caloric contents of the food they eat, a stunning 90 percent have no earthly idea how many calories they need in the first place. Studies have also shown that many people underestimate how many calories we take in, which means we think we're doing a good job, when in fact, we have a lot of work left to do.

Counting calories on the R3 Diet? The good news for you is that because you are eating four meals a day without getting seconds and on designated plates, you have halfway won the battle. I am not an advocate for obsessive calorie counting, but it is very beneficial to estimate your calories the first 30-days of your new eating plan. Why? Because if you are not aware of your basic calorie input, you could possibly put three handfuls of nuts on your salad meal, without the awareness that you just went over your daily caloric goal by 350 calories. On the other hand, if you had been doing quick estimates throughout the day of your four meals, you would have known to just add one handful of nuts to stay on target. By doing this for a solid month, you will have an idea of typical calories attached to many of your typical foods.

A portion of food is roughly equal to the size of your clenched fist or the palm of your hand. Each portion of protein or carbohydrate typically contains between 150 and 200 calories.

- Meat (one portion): 200 calories
- Potatoes (one baked): 200 calories
- Grains (one portion): 200 calories
- Handful of nuts (one portion): 175 calories
- Milk (one cup): 150 calories
- Creams, dressings and cheese sauce (one portion): 150 calories
- Beans (1portion): 125 calories
- Coconut Oil (1 Tbsp): 125 calories
- Fruit (one portion): 100 calories
- Bread (one slice, one tortilla): 100 calories
- Cheese (one cubic inch): 100 calories
- Butter (one pat): 100 calories
- Vegetables (one portion): 50 calories

Make sure to check the label or use an calorie counter website to check calories for a new food or recipe. It is also important that when you read the nutritional information on any food label, to be sure and check out what they call a serving.

What's the magical formula to achieve your weight goals?

In order for your weight to stay the same, the energy (or calories) you consume should equal the energy (or calories) you expend. In most cases, it's really a simple matter of energy balance: "Calories In" must equal "Calories Out." "Calories In" includes what we eat and drink. "Calories Out" includes our resting metabolic rate, thermic effect of food, and physical activity. Your personal calorie requirement depends on these three factors.

Calculate Your Total Calorie Needs

There are many equations to estimate your total calorie needs based on your RMR and level of physical activity (NOTE: the thermic effect of food is usually not accounted for since its role is so minor). It is important to realize that all these equations are just estimates. You may need more or less depending on genetic differences in RMR and your body composition.

Step 1: Estimate RMR

Men	**Healthy body weight x 11 calories**
Women	**Healthy body weight x 10 calories**

IMPORTANT NOTE: This is just an estimate of what your body requires *at rest*. If you have more muscle than the average person, you probably require *more* calories at rest than this equation suggests. If you have more fat than the average person, you probably require *fewer* calories at rest than this equation suggests. Remember, muscle mass is much more metabolically active than fat tissue. If you are 30 lbs. or more overweight (and that excess weight is mostly fat, not muscle), you can use your desired vs. actual body weight when calculating your RMR.

Step 2: Multiply RMR by Activity Factor

	Women	Men
Very Light/Sedentary (sitting or standing all day) e.g. lab/computer work, typing, painting	1.3	1.3
Light (walking and some movement throughout day) e.g. student, teacher, homemaker, child care worker	1.5	1.6
Moderate (job with some physical work or *moderate* intensity exercise 4-5 x/wk. for about one hour) e.g. gardening, carrying loads, most recreational exercisers	1.6	1.7

Heavy (job with heavy manual labor or *vigorous* intensity exercise 5-6 x/wk. for one or more hours) e.g. roofer, carpenter, many athletes	1.9	2.1
Exceptional (intense physical training for many hours every day) e.g. professional or collegiate athletes during their seasons	2.2	2.4

Shedding Fat

Step 3: Subtract 300-500 from your final number if your goal is to lose weight.

The only way to lose weight is to create a calorie deficit (either by eating fewer calories or burning more in physical activity). The *R3 Diet* will help you maximize fat loss, increase energy and increase the chances that you won't gain it back!

Note Calorie levels should never drop below 1200 calories per day for women or 1800 calories per day for men.

EATING JOURNALS

In a Kaiser Permanente Center for health study, dieters who kept track of what they ate in a daily food diary showed **double the weight loss** of those who didn't. This shows the power in this one underrated tool. "Those who kept daily food records lost twice as much weight as those who kept no records," lead author and Kaiser Permanente researcher Jack Hollis, PhD, told the press. "It seems that the simple act of writing down what you eat encourages people to consume fewer calories."

I have been sharing the results of that study with my clients for the past few years and have seen extraordinary results from the use of it. You can jot it on a pad of paper or in the notes section of your cell phone. Based on the benefits of food journaling, I have created the "R3 Journal" that is detailed and extremely efficient in helping you successfully follow the *R3 Diet*. It was designed to help you with the following:

- Food categories are listed to allow you to quickly put a dot next to the food.
- Fruits and vegetables are listed by colors to ensure variety.
- You can easily monitor calories to make sure you stay within your goal.
- The journal is reusable and easily portable and compact.
- It is a great grocery shopping guide.
- It helps you to become a conscious eater and establishes healthy eating habits.

Many people use it scrupulously for the first 30 days and then revisit it if they ever get off course, months or years later. Keeping things simple is the key. The R3 journal is simple to use with little time vested, yet power-packed in what it delivers. You can find out more on the R3 Journal at R3fitworld.com.

Supplements are my 3rd Pillar in my 4-pillar system. Remember that supplements fill in the cracks of what is missing in your eating. Obviously you do not need to take every supplement at the same time so the best way to structure supplementation is on a "perfect 7" in the form of daily's and rotations. Example: Your daily's are 1.Extra Virgin Coconut Oil, 2,Apple Cider Vinegar, 3.Multivitamin, 4.Antioxidant & 5.Chia Seeds #6 & #7 may change daily with supplements on your rotation shelf. Maybe you have magnesium, flax seeds, bee pollen, spirulina, l-glutamine, b12 & 5-HTP that you alternate in the that #6 & #7 spot.

CHAPTER 4

R U Ready for power-packed fuel?

15 Powerful Supplements

B-Complex is needed for the proper functioning of almost every process in the body. B Vitamins are water-soluble, which means any excess will be excreted through the urine. This also means that B Vitamins need to be taken on a daily basis, as the only one we can store is Vitamin B12.

B complex has a wide range of properties, including:

B1 (thiamine)—needed for release of energy from carbohydrates; aids in functioning of nervous system; helps maintain stomach acidity and normal appetite.

B2 (riboflavin)—needed for converting proteins, fats and carbo-hydrates into energy; necessary for healthy skin and eyes.

B3 (niacin)—needed for release of energy from food; maintains health of skin, mouth and digestive tract; necessary for normal mental function; can increase circulation and reduce high blood pressure.

B5 (pantothenic acid)—needed for release of energy from food; helps in the functioning of the adrenal gland and in the formation of antibodies.

B6 (pyridoxine)—needed for metabolism of protein, hence requirements related to protein intake; helps to maintain fluid balance, a requirement for healthy red blood cells.

B12—needed for red blood cell production and maintenance of protective sheath around nerves.

Folic acid—Essential for growth and reproduction of cells, particularly red blood cells.

Biotin—involved in carbohydrate, protein and fat metabolism. Also required for healthy skin and hair.

Flax contains lignans, which may have an antioxidant effect and block or suppress cancerous changes. Flax is also high in omega-3 fatty acids, which are thought to protect against colon cancer, breast cancer and heart disease. It also helps to reduce inflammation.

Hemp is one of the purest, most complete plants on earth. It has the perfect balance of Omega 3 and 6 for sustainable human health. This makes raw hemp seeds incredibly powerful against cancer. It might be the single best food to prevent it. It's a high quality, complete raw food protein and has a massive trace mineral content. It's the only seed that doesn't need to be germinated before eating: it has no enzyme exhibitors. Therefore it's easy to absorb. It also replenishes the muscles.

L-Glutamine powder prevents breakdown of muscle, brain and gut. It also stabilizes blood sugar.

Spirulina is green/blue algae powder, and has the highest concentration of nutrients known, including 60% protein content. It also helps control blood sugar and cravings. Spirulina and its relative, Chlorella, were introduced to the market in the 1970's. It is very popular among athletes and bodybuilders because it provides more stamina, strength and better nutrient absorption. It has a rich supply of bioavailable iron. Its many health benefits include immune system enhancement, anti-viral and cancer protective effect, reducing the harmful blood fats, reducing njurskadande effect of heavy metals and radiation protective effect. It has been tested in Japan and Europe and found to benefit people who suffer from many ailments including:

anemia, cataracts, diabetes, gastrointestinal disorders, glaucoma, hepatitis, and physical imbalances. Spirulina also aids in weight loss.

Chlorella gets its name from the high amount of chlorophyl it possesses. Chlorella contains more chlorophyl per gram than any other plant. Chlorophyl is one of the greatest food substances for cleansing the bowel and other elimination systems, such as the liver and the blood. It contains the widest range of essential nutrients available in any single food source, including potassium, all of the B vitamins, magnesium, zinc and iron, 18 vital amino acids, beta carotene and lutein.

Apple cider vinegar aids in digestion and the breakdown of fat. It neutralizes toxic substances, detoxifies blood and organs and prevents urine from becoming excessively alkaline.

Bee Pollen is esteemed by many health experts as a complete food. The bees pack the powder into granules, adding honey or nectar from honey sacs where it is then transported back to the hive. Finally, an enzyme is added to prevent germination, metabolizing the pollen for food, thus preserving the bee pollen benefit nutritionally. It helps with increasing energy and libido, helps eliminate acne, aids indigestion, eliminates depression, and improves blood pressure. Bee pollen contains many minerals including remarkably high levels of iron, zinc, manganese, and copper as well as potassium, calcium, and magnesium. It's also rich in most of the B vitamins and carotenes, which are the precursors of vitamin A.

Cayenne Pepper is a very high source of Vitamins A and C, has the complete B complexes, and is very rich in organic calcium and potassium, which is one of the reasons it is good for the heart. It significantly increases thermogenesis (heat production) and oxygen consumption for more than 20 minutes after it is eaten. The increase in oxygen during this time also causes you to burn more calories while also suppressing appetite. It is full of beta carotene and other antioxidants and immune boosters. It clears congestion and fights inflammation. Cayenne can rebuild the tissue in the stomach and aid the peristaltic action in the intestines.

Cinnamon stabilizes blood sugar, improves digestion and kills germs. When scientists added cinnamon to apple juice infected with a large amount of E.coli, the cinnamon destroyed more than 99% of the bacteria after three days at room temperature. Dr. Daniel Y.C. Fung, who supervised the apple juice research, thinks cinnamon has a bright future in germ fighting. "If cinnamon can knock out E.coli 0157:H7, one of the most virulent foodborne microorganisms that exists today," he says, "It will certainly have antimicrobial effects on other common foodborne bacteria, such as Salmonella and Campylobacter."

Digestive Enzymes are energized protein molecules essential for the digestion of food, brain stimulation, tissue, cell and organ repair; and generating cellular energy. Nutrients, including enzymes, work synergistically which means they cooperate with each other acting as catalysts. This promotes absorption and assimilation. The importance of digestive enzymes resides in the fact that the human body cannot absorb nutrients in food unless digestive enzymes break them down. The body progressively loses its ability to produce enzymes with major drops occurring roughly every ten years of life. At the beginning it may not be that noticeable, however, later on you will discover that you cannot tolerate or enjoy certain foods like you did before. This may also be accompanied by a feeling of reduced stamina. Yes, you're running low on enzymes. You will get lots of enzymes from your raw fruits and vegetables, but it would be wise to use a supplement before your "anything" meals.

Green Barley Grass: Barley grass, the green shoots of the barley, is reputed to be the only vegetation on earth that can supply sole nutritional support from birth to old age. Some of the vitamins in green barley grass are five B vitamins, including Vitamin B12. It also contains folic acid, panthothenic acid, B1, B2, B6, beta carotene, and C and E. And recent laboratory analysis on green barley grass has turned up traces of more than 70 minerals, among them calcium, iron, magnesium, and phosphorus.

Barley grass also contains 18 amino acids, which are the building blocks of proteins. Because barley green's proteins are polypeptides, or smaller proteins, they can be directly absorbed by the blood. Fresh barley grass is said to have thousands of active enzymes. Barley grass also contains chlorophyll. Green barley grass is also said to have a high alkalizing effect, because it contains the buffer minerals such as sodium, potassium, calcium and magnesium.

Extra virgin coconut oil: Approximately 50% of the fatty acids in coconut fat are lauric acid, the "good fat". Lauric acid is a medium chain fatty acid that supports healthy metabolism, which has the additional beneficial function of being formed into monolaurin in the human or animal body. Monolaurin is the antiviral, antibacterial, and antiprotozoal monoglyceride used by the human or animal to destroy lipid coated viruses helps increase metabolism and improve thyroid function and digestion. These fatty acids do not circulate in the bloodstream like other fats, but are sent directly to the liver where they are immediately converted into energy, just like carbohydrates. In this way, the body uses the fat in coconut oil to produce energy, rather than store it as body fat. Medium chain fatty acids found in coconut oil also speed up the body's metabolism, burning more calories and promoting weight loss. Other benefits include skin care, maintaining healthy cholesterol levels, losing weight, enhancing the immune system, maintaining a healthy heart, aiding proper digestion and robust metabolism, maintaining healthy blood pressure, diabetes and cancer prevention, increased energy, contributing to healthy teeth, hair, and bone strength. (More benefits of coconut oil listed previously)

Probiotics help the digestive system in many ways. They assist with digestion and help protect against harmful bacteria. They also help alleviate diarrhea, constipation and irritable bowel syndrome (IBS). Probiotics prevent and treat vaginal yeast infections and urinary tract infections, and reduce bladder cancer recurrence. They regulate immune function and shorten the duration of intestinal infections, and also prevent and treat inflammation following colon surgery, promoting anti-tumor and anti-cancer activity in the body. Probiotics also increase the body's ability to synthesize vitamin B and absorb calcium, assimilate the nutrients from food and help to reduce lactose intolerance.

Wheatgrass stimulates the metabolism and the body's enzyme systems by enriching the blood. It also aids in reducing blood pressure by dilating the blood pathways throughout the body. It stimulates the thyroid gland, correcting obesity, indigestion, and a host of other complaints. Wheatgrass is also a beauty treatment that slows down the aging process.

15 Powerful Super foods

Superfoods are foods that are said to have more nutrients and unique properties than typical foods. They can sometimes be foods with a high phytonutrient content. ALL fruits and vegetables are heroes but let's take a look at some of the characteristics of the super-heroes.

Avocados were once outlawed on diets for their fat content; however the avocado has made the list for its high levels of fiber, vitamins C and B6, and folate. Avocados have "healthy" fats that lower LDL cholesterol levels ("bad" cholesterol) and raise HDL cholesterol levels ("good" cholesterol).

Bananas contain many properties to put them on the super-food list. Because of their abundance of vitamins and minerals, bananas are a great source of natural energy. They neutralize the acidity of gastric juices, thus reducing ulcer irritation by coating the lining of the stomach. Not only can bananas relieve painful systems of ulcers and other intestinal disorders, they can also promote healing. Their high iron content helps to cure anemia, and they stimulate the production of hemoglobin in the blood. Bananas are known for promoting healthy digestion and creating a feeling of youthfulness. They promote healthy bones by helping the body absorb calcium. Bananas are high in B vitamins, vitamin C, iron and magnesium. Most importantly relating to exercise, bananas contain high levels of potassium, which enables muscles to contract and expand smoothly as well as reduce cramping. Bananas might also help individuals with depression due to their tryptophan content, which is believed to increase serotonin levels in the brain.

Beans (dried and green) and lentils are extremely fibrous energy stabilizers; Beans also contain isoflavones, which studies show can reduce cancer risk. Beans contain vitamin B and potassium and as much cholesterol-lowering fiber as oats.

Beets contain a pigment that gives them their super-beautiful fuschia color. This pigment, known as betacyanin, is also a powerful cancer-fighting agent. Beets' potential effectiveness against colon cancer, in particular, has been demonstrated in several studies. Beets are also particularly rich in the B vitamin folate.

Berries pack an incredible amount of nutritional goodness into a small package. They're loaded with antioxidants and phytonutrients, are low in calories, high in water and fiber content, which help control blood sugar and keep you feeling full longer. Their flavors satisfy sweets cravings for a fraction of the calories found in baked goods. Blueberries lead the pack because they are among the best source of antioxidants and are widely available. Cranberries are also widely available and good for you because they are packed with antioxidants, have the ability to prevent urinary tract infections. They also lower harmful cholesterol (LDL) while raising good cholesterol (HDL) in the body.

Carrots slow aging, promote healthy vision, have anti-cancer properties, and increase immunity towards various chronic diseases. Yes, carrots do it all for you! This natural health booster enhances your health on various grounds and fills in the essential vitamins to your body like pro-vitamin A, B3, C and E. Other important advantages of carrots include preventing various gastrointestinal complaints like colic and ulcers. Their high soluble fiber content also helps to prevent heart attacks and cancer by reducing cholesterol.

Cherries are rich in antioxidants that help to prevent cancer and protect the body from the damage caused by free radicals. Cherries can reduce pain and inflammation from arthritis and gout while also helping to promote weight loss. They help prevent diabetes, heart disease, and memory loss, and lower cholesterol levels. Studies suggest the quercetin found in cherries is a natural anti-inflammatory and source of energy, and may help to relieve symptoms of depression and anxiety. Both sweet and sour cherries are a rich source of vitamin C, which helps boost immunity, lower the risk of stroke and improve the overall look of skin by reducing the appearance of wrinkles and dry skin. The vitamin C works together with the anthocyanins, and proanthocyanidins found in cherries to strengthen collagen, which helps strengthen joints and muscles. The melatonin in cherries may promote better sleep for those who experience insomnia.

Durian is an Asian fruit containing phytonutrients that provide immune system support, blood detoxification, and powerful antioxidant and anti-inflammatory effects. It has minerals such as calcium, iron, magnesium, phosphorus, potassium, sodium, zinc, copper and manganese. Its vitamin content includes thiamin, riboflavin, niacin, vitamin A, vitamins B5 and B6, vitamin C, folic acid and retinol. Also compared to other fruits, it is exceptionally high in protein and fat and is 100% cholesterol free. In Southeast Asia, durian is known as the "King of Fruits".

Guava is hailed by some researchers as the most nutritious fruit. Guavas are high in dietary fiber, vitamins A and C, vitamin B3 and G4 and polyunsaturated fatty acids, especially the seeds. It has four times the amount of vitamin C in oranges, contains excellent levels of the dietary minerals potassium and magnesium, as well as an otherwise broad, low-calorie profile of essential nutrients. Guavas contain both major classes of antioxidant pigments—carotenoids and polyphenols. Guavas that are red, yellow or orange in color have more potential value as antioxidant sources than unpigmented species.

Kale is a leafy green vegetable that belongs to the Brassica family, a group of vegetables including cabbage, collard greens and Brussels sprouts that are healthy additions to your plate. Kale is high in vitamins A and C and contains moderate amounts of calcium and other minerals. It is rich in antioxidants, especially the carotenoid beta carotene. In fact, kale has the highest Oxygen Radical Absorbance Capacity (ORAC) score—a measure of the total amount of antioxidants in a food—of any vegetable. It's great for your eyes, bones and skin.

Plums are packed with vitamins, simply put. Part of the peach and cherry family of fruits, they contain vitamins A, K, C, B6 and E, plus niacin, riboflavin, thiamin, pantothenic acid, and folate. It is one of those fruits that are rich in dietary fiber, which in turn improves the digestive system. The vitamin C and phenols in plums have antioxidant qualities, which look after the eyes and prevent macular degeneration, boost immunity, improve cardiac health and body tissue, and protect against cancer. Plums are in fact rich in antioxidants, which provide protection from the superoxide anion radical These antioxidants also prevent damage to our neurons and the fats that are part of our cell membranes. Plums also lead to better absorption of iron, and have strong antibacterial properties. They help regenerate the cells after heavy physical exercise or mental fatigue. The vitamin C in plums helps prevent flu and colds and stop cholesterol from getting oxidized. By neutralizing the free radicals, it prevents diseases like rheumatoid arthritis, osteoarthritis, colon cancer and asthma. And last but not least, plums have a positive cosmetic impact upon the skin.

Pomegranates offer very high antioxidant activity like brain and memory protection. Research has shown that drinking pomegranate juice may help lower the risk hardening of the arteries or atherosclerosis.

Quinoa [pronounced KEEN-wah], a member of the grain family, is considered a "complete" protein, which means that it packs all of the essential amino acids your body needs to build muscle.

Sweet potatoes are a delicious member of the dark orange vegetable family, which lead the pack in vitamin A content. It's also loaded with vitamin C, calcium, and potassium. Other dark orange vegetable standouts include pumpkin, carrots, butternut squash, and orange bell peppers.

Tomatoes contain a wide variety of nutrient and non-nutrient components, including lycopene, vitamins C, A and K, potassium, and fiber. One medium-sized tomato may provide almost half of a person's recommended daily amount of vitamin C. Various tomato components are believed to work together to produce health benefits. These include aiding in the development of healthy teeth, bones, skin and hair; lowering blood pressure and cholesterol levels and possibly reducing the risk of cardiovascular disease and some cancers.

Seaweeds: The following chart lists some of the more common edible seaweeds, their description, nutrients they contain and their most common uses.

Common Name	Description	Nutrients	Uses
Arame	dark thread like shapes; probably the most mild & tastiest variety	calcium, iron, iodine and protein	steamed, sautéed, added to soups & salads
Dulse	reddish-purple leafy; rinse thoroughly to remove some of the strong taste	protein, iron, fluoride, potassium, iodine and phosphorous, and vitamins B6 and B12.	eaten directly as seaweed "chips" or added to soups, sauces, salads, and relishes
Hijiki	black, sold dried in short course strips; Slightly bitter tasting	iron, protein, calcium, zinc and iodine	best used in dishes that require slow cooking
Kelp	Dried kelp swells to twice its volume when wet. (3) Before using, soak fronds in fresh water for two days	higher in iodine and potassium than the other sea vegetables high in calcium, potassium, magnesium, iron, and trace minerals	eaten fresh-chopped, added to a salad, sun-dried and crumbled as a salt substitute, good for soup stocks. Leave it in to "dissolve," for approximately ½ hour, or take it out after 15 minutes. A slab of kelp in any bean-based dish will enrich digestibility and shorten cooking time

Kombu	brown seaweed regarded as delicacies and sold for high prices	is meatier and also higher in sodium	good in soups and bean dishes to cut down on the gas producing enzymes
Nori/ Laverbread	A Japanese red seaweed, looks blackish in tins and when dried in sheets; also picked on the rugged coastline of Wales	high protein content (25-35% of dry weight), and is also high in vitamin A, calcium and iron, vitamin C content is about 1.5 times that of oranges	used in soups, as a seasoning for many dishes, commonly used as a wrapping for sushi, also added to cheeses
Wakame	brown seaweed regarded as delicacies and sold for high prices	is meatier and also higher in sodium	good in soups and added to bean dishes to cut down on the gas producing enzymes

CHAPTER 5

R U thirsty?

Beverages—some are good, some are not.

Water: Water is the essence of life and is needed by every cell in your body. Approximately 60%-70% of your body is made up of water. Water is an essential nutrient. All chemical reactions in the body depend upon it. If you're trying to lose weight, this can't be ignored. You won't be able to lose weight without water to flush out the by-products of fat breakdown. When there isn't enough water to dilute the body's waste products, kidney stones may form. When the kidneys aren't working to their full potential, the liver must step in and help. Once this happens the liver can't optimally perform its other important functions. As a result, burning fat has to wait.

Water helps to maintain proper muscle tone by giving muscles their natural ability to contract and by preventing dehydration. It also helps to prevent the sagging skin that usually follows weight loss—shrinking cells are buoyed by water which plumps the skin and leaves it clear, healthy and resilient.

Water plays a key role in the prevention of disease.

When the skin is properly hydrated, it looks plump and more radiant. Water will keep the toxins flushed out and help you to cool off through perspiration. More benefits include increased energy, more life vitality, ongoing detox, glowing and clearer skin, better digestion, better concentration, less painful menstruation, good regular bowel movements and many more!

We all know in economics what happens with a big demand and a small supply—economic upheaval. The body experiences a similar upheaval—of the digestive kind.

Wake up to water! As soon as you wake up, drink one to four eight-ounce glasses of room-temperature water **through a straw**. If you drink water from a glass or a bottle, you consume mostly air and feel bloated from all the air in your stomach. When you drink through a straw, you consume 95 percent water. You can drink four times as much before you feel full. Add two teaspoons of freshly squeezed lemon or lime juice to your water three times a day: upon rising, mid-afternoon, and in your final water intake in the evening. The juice will help alkalize your body and neutralize acids created from digesting certain foods or normal cellular metabolism.

Although you should not drink immediately before you eat, water intake should precede food intake by half an hour. Having one to two, eight-ounce glasses of water through a straw is optimal. If you do not have enough water in your stomach, digestion is impaired. Also, if the blood becomes too thick after eating because of lack of water, the blood will try to draw water from the cells. If you exercise or work hard and sweat in hot weather, add four eight-ounce glasses of water per hour of strenuous exercise or work. (This is the only time where it is best to drink your water cold) If you are trying to lose weight, you'll want to know that water suppresses the appetite naturally and helps the body metabolize stored fat.

Never drink while you are eating. The liquid flushes through the stomach quickly into the small intestine. It will dilute and drain some of the digestive juices out of the stomach. This spells stress, as the body must secrete more digestive enzymes. If you continue to consume liquid while you eat, your body's signals get confused. The stomach says, "Quick, there are no enzymes. Secrete more." The body says, "What's wrong? Just sent some!" (If you get thirsty during meals take a few sips of water only.)

Wait a half an hour after any meal to drink water. This holds true especially at supper, when consuming your last water of the evening. Fresh fruit juices or vegetable juices count as a glass of water, as do unsweetened herbal teas. Besides being good sources of vitamins, minerals and fiber, fruits and vegetables actually contain great amounts of water. If you eat a lot of water-rich fresh fruits and vegetables, they will easily provide you with two or three eight-ounce glasses.

Milk

What if all this dirt about dairy was just a bad dream?

The milk marketing boards would love for you to wake up to that unreality. But it's the producers of *organic* milk and dairy who just might have a case. Writes Ontario naturopath and organic dairy farmer John Pronk:

> The raging debate over 'milk as medicine' vs. 'milk as poison' reflects how today's food processing techniques can completely alter the state of a food, changing it from its natural healthy form to something totally different," "Modern processing techniques (pasteurizing, homogenizing, and skimming) destroy most of the beneficial nutrients in milk. Enzymes (which make milk easy to digest) and beneficial bacteria (which prevent people from developing allergies to foods) present in raw milk are destroyed by the heat of pasteurization, making it harder to digest and more allergenic.

> Dairy cattle are now fed a fixed ration of feeds which they would not typically eat if given a choice . . . . Not only might this be considered inhumane, but what is not considered is the effect of these feeds on the quality of the milk and the effects of this milk on those who drink it.

Having to deal with feeds that disagree puts an extra stress on a cow's immune system. Stressed cows are much more susceptible to infections and, not surprisingly, farmers are seeing very high rates of mastitis (udder infection) in these herds. The typical treatment for mastitis is antibiotics; antibiotic residues then end up in the milk. Overuse of these antibiotics has lead to the problem of antibiotic resistance.

Milk has historically been used very effectively as medicine for a number of different conditions. Fresh raw milk from healthy animals contains many beneficial nutrients that can be very nourishing and healing. Complete protein, lactoferrin, various digestive enzymes, immunoglobulins (antibodies), conjugated linoleic acid (CLA), and beneficial lactobacillus bacteria are just a few of the valuable nutrients that milk, in its natural form, supplies . . . .

I would say that organic milk is a lot closer to the whole food milk used to be. I would consider conventional store-bought milk to be a 'modified milk ingredient'; nothing close to the natural food it was a century ago.

Although the healthfulness and medicinal value of organic milk is still more a matter of lore than science, one thing is for sure: the evidence against modern milk can no more be applied to organic milk than the evidence against white rice can be applied to brown. These are cows of an entirely different color.

When choosing milk/dairy is it best to choose low-fat/fat free or full fat? Choose full fat because the fat is needed to absorb vitamins A, K, E and D, and calcium, so skim and low-fat milk do not provide any similar assimilation or protection. Likewise, fortified products are not the same at all. The fat is where the medium-chain triglycerides, *butyric acid*, omega-3 fatty acids and conjugated linoleic acid are located. The fat is often replaced with chemicals or sugar to make it more palatable and attractive. Heat alters milk's amino acids lysine and tyrosine making the proteins less available which promotes the rancidity of unsaturated fatty acids and destruction of vitamins. There is a loss of the anti stiffness factor and B12. The process puts an unnecessary strain on the pancreas to produce digestive enzymes.

Are there any more healthy milk options? Goat's milk!!! I give this to my kids because it is the closest to mother's milk than any other food. It has superior digestibility. It is a medium chain fatty acid. It is a complete protein (amino acid). It is rich in vitamin A and 30% of the daily calcium requirement.

Our body needs calcium, sooooo . . . . . what are some of the best non-milk sources for calcium-rich foods? Green leafy vegetables, bok choy, collard greens, kale, parsley, oranges, sesame seeds, broccoli, almonds, figs, and carrots. The optimal amount of calcium the average person needs is 500 to 700 mg /day. A cup of broccoli yields 178mg of calcium *NOTE: Salt and caffeine reduce calcium absorption.

Coffee

One cup of coffee contains between 65-100mg of caffeine. Caffeine has many detrimental effects to the body, some of which are: adrenal exhaustion, nausea, heart palpitations, dehydration, heartburn, insomnia, migraines, anxiety, bladder and kidney irritation and constipation. Coffee may also increase the risk of osteoporosis and hypertension if over-consumed. Clinical Nutritionist Stephen Cherniske wrote a book on the subject, "Caffeine Blues..Wake Up to the Hidden Dangers of America's #1 Drug" and it seems to be the most revealing and eye-opening tome on the topic. Many of the following statements are from his book.

Caffeine is produced by more than eighty species of plants. The reason may well be survival. As it turns out, caffeine is a biological poison used by plants as a pesticide.

Only 1% of caffeine is excreted within several hours after consumption. The remaining 99% has to be detoxified by the liver.

It can take up to 12 hours to detoxify a **single** cup of coffee.

Caffeine does not give you energy. It stimulates your nervous system and adrenals. That's not energy, that's stress.

Not only is caffeine addictive, it also encourages other addictions to substances like nicotine.

DHEA is our vitality hormone. Decreased levels of DHEA is a cause of aging. Caffeine consumption leads to DHEA deficiency. Caffeine is an AGING DRUG!

Caffeine lowers the stress threshold in virtually everyone. That is, if you have had caffeine, it will be easier for you to suffer from emotional stress or other stress.

Caffeine disrupts sleep. Deep sleep is CRITICAL to good health. When there's caffeine in your bloodstream, you are unlikely to experience deep sleep at all!

Malnutrition is one of the most well-defined effects of habitual caffeine intake.

A single cup of coffee can reduce iron absorption from a meal by as much as 75%.

People do not develop a tolerance to the anxiety-producing effects of caffeine. Rather, people simply become accustomed to the feelings of stress, irritability and aggressiveness produced by the drug.

Caffeine contributes to depression in well-defined ways. This is particularly due to the withdrawal effect, which can cause headache, depression and fatigue, even in light users. Cherniske reported that 90% of people who came to him suffering from depression and gave up caffeine completely for two months reported that their depression went away!

Caffeine depletes your supplies of thiamin and other B vitamins, calcium, magnesium, potassium, iron and zinc.

Caffeine increases calcium loss and risk of osteoporosis.

Caffeine DOES NOT improve learning or memory. In fact the exact opposite is true. Scientific studies have shown that caffeine as normally consumed can reduce cerebral flow by as much as 30%. That means less oxygen to the brain and reduced memory and cognition.

Caffeine is also a major cause of heart attacks and cancer. If the withdrawal symptoms you get from letting go of caffeine do not let you know that it is detrimental to your health, then I don't know what does.

Coffee is the largest agricultural commodity in the world. More coffee is grown and traded than wheat rice, corn or livestock. More than fruit, vegetables or any staple of the diet, COFFEE is number one. In fact, it's the third leading commodity after petroleum and strategic metals. That's more than automobiles, steel, and technology. Add those three together and it still couldn't touch coffee. Why? *Because coffee is addictive.*

There's another problem. Coffee is also the most heavily sprayed of all agricultural commodities. It is grown in regions where there are very few restrictions, regulations or protections regarding pesticide use. The environmental impact is tremendous.

Regular and Diet Sodas

Soda has an alarming amount of sugar, calories and harmful additives in it that have absolutely no nutritional value. Soda comprises more than one-fourth of all drinks that are consumed in the United States. There is also a direct link between tooth decay and soft drinks. The high acid levels in all sodas dissolve the calcium out of the enamel, leaving a softened matrix for bacteria to enter the teeth and cause cavities. Sodas are also a major source of caffeine (see caffeine effects above).

You may have heard of a chemical called aspartame, which is used as a sugar substitute in diet soda. There are over 92 different health side effects associated with aspartame consumption , including brain tumors, birth defects, diabetes, emotional disorders and epilepsy/seizures. Further, when aspartame is stored for long periods of time or kept in warm areas it changes to methanol, an alcohol that itself converts to formaldehyde and formic acid, which are known carcinogens.

"In animal studies, giving them small quantities of artificial sweeteners over a couple of weeks leads to a small but statistically significant increase of body weight gain," says Susan Swithers, a psychologist at Purdue University's Ingestive Behavior Research Center. That may be because the body associates sweetness with calorie intake, and when one eats something sweet, the body prepares for an increase in calories. When those calories don't come, the body gets confused-which could lead to a slowing of metabolism or a craving for more food to offset the perceived loss. Please realize that you DO NOT lose weight from drinking diet soda, it is the exact opposite.

Energy Drinks

Energy drinks are marketed as all-natural energy boosters loaded with exotic ingredients that popular culture believes to be healthy. They are typically marketed toward younger crowds. In 2006 young adults spent almost $2.3 billion on energy drinks—money that could be put to better use on more important things than a sugary energy beverage. Energy drinks contain two main ingredients: caffeine and sugar. The drinks do basically what they say—give their drinkers an energy boost. Energy drink labels are frequently misleading or at least so ambiguous that when you buy them you simply believe what you want to believe. A typical energy drink can contain up to 80 milligrams of sugar. Energy drinks are addicting because they have extremely high amounts of caffeine. A typical 16-ounce can of your average energy drink has 160 milligrams of caffeine. Many energy drinks have a high sodium content as well. These have the same negative side effects as coffee.

Fortified Waters/Low Calorie Powdered Drink Mixes/Sports Drinks

These can all be summed up by the following statement: The beverage industry is a billion dollar industry that stays strong by knowing that you want to "feel" health conscious and selling you glorified sugar water that has healthy buzz words on the label.

CHAPTER 6

R U Ready for the dangers?

Sugar

The United States Department of Agriculture (USDA) reports that the average American consumes anywhere between *150 to 170 pounds of sugar per year!*

An average American consumes more than fifty pounds of artificial sweeteners per year.

Even if you don't indulge in dessert foods, the carbohydrates from heavily processed, nutrient-deficient breads, crackers, and chips of all kinds will have exactly the same effect as sugar.

Our bodies crave sugar naturally, but it is meant for us to reach for fresh fruit. There is nothing wrong with the prompting, but there is a huge problem with what we are reaching for. When you eat a lot of sugar your body over-produces the hormone insulin. The insulin reacts with the sugar, causing blood sugar to drop. When your blood sugar drops, you crave more sugar. This is the cycle of sugar addiction. Of all the foods consumed today, refined sugar is considered to be one of the most harmful.

Refined sugar contains no fiber, no minerals, no proteins, no fats, no enzymes; only empty calories. What happens when you eat a refined carbohydrate like sugar? Your body must borrow vital nutrients from healthy cells to metabolize the incomplete food. Calcium, sodium, potassium and magnesium are taken from various parts of the body to make use of the sugar. Oftentimes, so much calcium is used to neutralize the effects of sugar that the bones become osteoporotic due to the withdrawn calcium. (Hence, once again, the catastrophic levels of osteoporosis in western countries like the U.S.)

All of the following are the effects of sugar on the body:

Heart disease from raised blood triglycerides and sticky blood platelets

Duodenal ulcers from increased stomach acidity

Hypoglycemia

Increase in the amount of food that you eat

Diabetes

Hyperactivity

Liver enlargement

Kidney enlargement

Indigestion

Headaches and migraines

Increased fat storage

Sex hormone imbalance

Increase in uric acid in blood

Cancer

Hindered breakdown of dietary protein

Cavities

Calcium leached from teeth

Collagen damage, leading to wrinkles and skin aging

Slowdown in adrenal gland function

Can be intoxicating, similar to alcohol

Reduces learning capacity

Weakened immune system

PMS

Yeast overgrowth

Excessive and/or foul-smelling intestinal gas

Sugar dependency

Flu-like symptoms

Varicose veins

Upset stomach

Can lead to alcoholism

Irritability
Manic-depressive tendencies

Can cause a decrease in insulin sensitivity

Chronic or frequent bouts of depression

Can increase cholesterol

Difficulty concentrating

Induces salt and water retention

Forgetfulness or absentmindedness

Intense sleepiness not caused by lack of sleep

Lack of motivation

Muscle fatigue

Increased undependability

Lethargy

Loss of enthusiasm for plans and projects

Pallor

Inconsistency in thoughts and actions

Coated tongue and persistent thirstiness

Situational personality changes

Bad breath

Irrational thoughts

Heartburn/sour stomach

Emotional outbursts

Chromium deficiency.

Eating disorders

Snacking

A snack is anything consumed between your meals. 60% of Americans eat snack food regularly, consuming about 20% of their calories from snacks. Since snacking in between meals is not allowed on the *R3 Diet*, you will find that you put more time, appreciation and thought into your meals. Snacking is the thorn in every diet. It causes you to always be snacking on something or looking for something to snack on. They don't fill you up and typically just add extra, unnecessary calories to your day. Snacking is an unnecessary and destructive habit. Well, you may ask, what about "healthy" snacks? My response is to put the thought into healthy meals that keep you nourished and satiated until the next meal.

Binge Eating

Binge eating disorder is a newly recognized condition that affects millions of Americans. People with binge eating disorder frequently eat large amounts of food while feeling a loss of control over their eating. New research suggests that binge eating is the most common type of eating disorder. This disorder is different from binge-purge syndrome (bulimia nervosa) because people with binge eating disorder usually do not purge afterward by vomiting or using laxatives. Most of us overeat from time to time, and many people feel they frequently eat more than they should. Eating large amounts of food, however, does not mean that a person has binge eating disorder. But most people with serious binge eating problems have:

- Frequent episodes of eating what others would consider an abnormally large amount of food.
- Frequent feelings of being unable to control what or how much is being eaten.
- Several of the following behaviors or feelings:

  1. Eating much more rapidly than usual
  2. Eating until uncomfortably full

3. Eating large amounts of food, even when not physically hungry
4. Eating alone out of embarrassment at the quantity of food being eaten
5. Feelings of disgust, depression, or guilt after overeating

A survey published in *Biological Psychiatry* (Feb 1 2007, vol. 61) found that people struggle with symptoms of binge eating for an average of eight years before seeking treatment. As a binge eater, you feel hopeless because the feeling to keep eating seems unstoppable. Each time you do it, you convince yourself that it will be your last. You feel that you are not exhibiting enough will power. You feel like others enjoy their meals and move on throughout their day, while you are stuck feeling obsessed, overpowered and overconsumed with thoughts and food. Have you ever felt like you were addicted to certain foods? You know the feeling. You pop a candy in your mouth and you're off and running on a binge. You can't have just one chip or a serving of ice cream. One taste and you eat a mountain of it. Or, you're doing really well on your healthier lifestyle journey and then one day you decide to stray a bit.

Perhaps you're stressed out or maybe you thought "Hey, I've been doing really well and I feel like taking a 'vacation day' from my program to eat whatever I like." And then you have that piece of cake or cookie and even after gulping down everything in sight, it's still not enough.

Here's the good news. You're not crazy. You could be addicted. Researchers at the Scripps Research Institute have just published a study that explains why you eat so compulsively around particular foods. You may actually be a *junk food* junkie!

This exciting new study was funded by the National Institute of Drug Abuse, a department of the National Institutes of Health (NIH). Since drug addiction and obesity are major national problems, researchers set out to see if brain changes that take place in drug addiction were present in the obese. Prior studies have shown that both drug addiction and obesity were associated with a dysfunction in the brain's reward system. The more you indulge in drugs or sugary-fatty foods, the higher your reward threshold and the more you want. It becomes a vicious cycle of trying to curb a craving that can never be fully satisfied.

In this study, one group of rats was fed a normal diet with limited access to junk food. They gained some weight but did not become obese. The other group of rats was also fed their usual food but was allowed unlimited exposure to real junk food, including candy, cake, bacon, sausage and more. Over time, the rats were observed to find the junk food tasty, and their consumption continued to increase, resulting in obesity.

(What was really interesting was the fact that the rats kept coming back for more despite the fact that electric shocks were administered to them if they did. You might recall a time when you braved snow, sleet, and pouring rain to get to the store to satisfy your craving for candy, ice cream, pizza, chips or some other snack food. We'll do anything to scratch that addictive itch, won't we?)

Now for the coup de grace. After 40 days, the researchers took all of the junk food away and replaced it with the normal healthy rat food. Guess what? The obese rats went on a hunger strike for two weeks and refused to eat it. Hah! That's like being forced to go on a "diet" when all you can think of is scoring food for your next binge. Eventually the rats settled down and reluctantly shed pounds as they acclimated to their usual food. But I'll guarantee you if those snacks are placed in the cage two months from now, the rats will reawaken those taste memories in a heartbeat.

So what gives? What is happening here? The researchers found that special dopamine receptors (dopamine is the 'pleasure' brain neurotransmitter) became suppressed as the rats became more obese. The reward system, in essence, had begun to deteriorate. The rats began to eat compulsively, desperately seeking the taste reward they craved, only to find that it took more and more junk food to achieve the goal.

This is exactly what happens to humans addicted to cocaine or heroin. Other studies have noted that certain foods can be addictive.

Rush University researchers have found that these foods include sweets, sweet/fat combos, and potentially processed and salty foods. Sounds like the usual binge foods.

What does all of this mean to you? Well, you might just be wiping the shock right off your face. You've known intuitively that certain foods are nothing but binging trouble and so you steer clear. You'll probably also notice that it's never tuna on a bed of greens or pears that gets you going. Instead it is, as science has shown, refined sugars, high fats and processed foods that will set you off into an addictive compulsive eating craze.

Here are some tips from Pamela Peeke, MD, MPH, FACP to help you navigate the treacherous waters of addictive eating:

1. **Make a list of any foods that lead to overeating and/or binging.** You know what they are. Some are sweet eaters, others like starches; still more have problems with both. Sit down and write them out. Be aware and keep these foods out of your house and stay away from them at restaurants and social gatherings.

2. **Do not fall for the "just one little bite" lie.** It's like an alcoholic's "just one little drink" rationalizing. Don't try it. You'll lose every time. If it's an addictive food, your having even a small amount may awaken the beast and set you off on a regrettable binge.

3. **Get the right attitude.** You're not being deprived of a tasty delight. You're saving yourself from a shame and guilt-filled binge, and all those extra pounds of body fat.

4. **Summon a support team.** If you're really having issues with these foods, then put together your own A-Team. You can draw upon people who show compassion and want to support your efforts to withdraw from these foods. Family, friends, expert counselors, medical and fitness professionals, dietitians and groups like *Overeaters Anonymous* may be good resources.

5. **Be patient and persistent.** You need to give your body enough time to adapt and adjust to healthier foods. Even the rats needed two weeks to get over their food strike! Keep plenty

of fresh produce and lean protein around and plan your meals and snacks so you're not left in the lurch with only the addictive stuff to choose. You can do this!

Well I am speaking from an intimately close experience when I say that it can be overcome; I repeat, it CAN be overcome. The *R3 Diet* is designed with binge eating in mind and if you follow it precisely, you will kiss binge eating goodbye in weeks. I speak for myself and many others when I say that it is an amazing feeling when you go from living to eat, to **eating to live.**

Elimination

What exactly is constipation? Constipation is a common digestive problem. It may be difficult for you to have a bowel movement, or your bowel movements may be infrequent. You may be getting constipated if you start having bowel movements much less often than you usually do. As the food you eat passes through your digestive tract, your body takes nutrients and water from the food. This process creates a stool, which is moved through your intestines with muscle contractions (squeezing motions). A number of things can affect this process. These include not drinking enough fluids, not being active enough, not eating enough fiber or produce, as well as taking certain medicines. If you eat three meals a day, then you should have three bowel movements each day. The first bowel movement should take place in the morning when you wake up or soon after you have had breakfast. Typically you should experience the urge for a bowel movement 20-30 minutes after you eat. The other bowel movements should be during the day and just before bedtime.

In her book, *Healthy Digestion the Natural Way* (2000), D. Lindsey Berkson defines constipation, "A healthy person should have at least one bowel movement a day. Medical textbooks state that individual variation goes from several times a day to several times a week. However, having worked with people for many years on improving their health, I would define constipation as not having one to several daily bowel movements, or having too long an intestinal-transit time."

If you eat three meals a day and only have one or two bowel movements, then the second and third meals are backing up in your colon and staying there too long. When your fecal matter stays too long in your colon, water and toxins are pulled out of the fecal matter and absorbed through your colon wall. This makes the fecal matter stiff and hard. Your colon will now have a hard time moving this hard fecal matter through its sections and out the rectum.

Foods rich in fiber will help to regulate the digestive system. These include:

- Unprocessed wheat bran
- Unrefined breakfast cereals
- Whole-grain bread and brown rice
- Fresh fruits
- Dried fruits (such as prunes, apricots and figs)
- Vegetables
- Beans (such as navy, kidney and pinto beans)

CHAPTER 7

R U Ready for the cleansers?

Juice Fasting

Juice fasting is the oldest, fastest, least expensive and most effective healing method known to humankind, with more testimonials from our greatest thinkers and spiritual teachers than all other healing modalities combined. Unfortunately, today's mostly Western diets are heavily loaded with artificial flavors and chemically-created coloring agents, toxic pesticides, herbicides, fungicides, insecticides, and other toxic chemicals which overburden our bodies. As this toxic overload accumulates decade after decade, augmented by environmental pollution, drugs and medications, it eventually interferes with normal functioning and our body's elimination becomes impaired.

During fasting, large amounts of these accumulated metabolic wastes and poisons are very quickly eliminated through the greatly enhanced cleansing capability of all the organs of elimination—liver, kidneys, skin and lungs. Several common symptoms of detoxification seen during this process could be darker urine, which signals the possibility of catarrhal elimination of excess mucus. During fasting, your body will "autolyze", or self-digest, its most inferior and impure materials and metabolic wastes, including: fat deposits, abscesses, dead and dying cells, bumps and protuberances, damaged tissue, calluses, furuncles (small skin abscesses, or boils), morbid accumulations, growths, and amazingly, various kinds of neoplasms (abnormal growths of tissue, or tumors). German and Swedish biological clinics, operated by medical doctors, routinely treat nearly every disease, from cardiovascular and digestive disorders to rheumatic and skin conditions, with scientific, therapeutic fasting. Germany's late Otto Buchinger,Sr., M.D., supervised over 100,000 successful "juice fasting cures." In Russia, fasting has been used for over a half-century as the most effective treatment for schizophrenia, with irrefragable studies showing that 70% of patients improved mentally after 20-to-30 days of controlled fasting. Similarly, one Japanese research clinic fasted 382 patients, all suffering psychosomatic disease, with a success rate of 87%.

North America is still far behind the learning curve, nevertheless, as is clear to Dr. Charles Goodrich of the Mt. Sinai School of Medicine in New York City, who has fasted countless times. "People don't realize that the chief obstacle to fasting is overcoming the cultural, social and psychological fears of going without food," he says, "These fears are ingrained . . . . However, fasting is not starving, not even in a medical sense or the natural sense." Dr. George Cahill of Harvard Medical School emphasized the point. "Man's survival [of long abstentions from food] is predicated upon a remarkable ability to conserve the relatively limited body protein stores, while utilizing fat as the primary energy producing food." In *Fasting and Eating for Health*, Joel Fuhrman, M.D., notes, (p. 10): "The fast does not merely detoxify; it also breaks down superfluous tissue—fat, abnormal cells, athermanous plaque, and tumors—and releases diseased tissues and their cellular products into the circulation for elimination. Toxic or unwanted materials circulate in our bloodstream and lymphatic tissues, and are deposited in and released from our fat stores and other tissues. An important element of fasting detoxification is mobilizing the toxins from their storage areas."

An important component to a successful juice fast is a reliable machine. A juice extractor is able to extract 70% to 98% of the nutrients from vegetables. When you pass a vegetable through the juice machine, it effectively separates the juice that is locked in the fibers. By drinking the juice, the majority of nutrients are absorbed directly into the bloodstream without the work of digestion. An abundant supply of nutrients in conjunction with minimum digestive effort is a perfect healing environment. Bodily energy normally involved in your mastication, assimilation, digestion, and elimination is freed up. This is another reason you'll feel more—not less—energy throughout properly-done juice fasting. The main difference in juicing versus smoothies is the fiber content. Fiber is good during eating but not when you are fasting. When you juice you withhold the fiber.

What should I do first?

Start a raw-foods diet seven days prior to juice fasting. Eliminate ALL caffeine, sweets, refined foods and junk foods a week prior and through your juice fast.

What will I need?

A juicer (which can range from $60 to over $300). Great lower-end juicers are the Jack LaLanne Power Juicer and Juiceman brands. Great higher-end juicer brands are Champion and Breville. Use fresh, preferably organic vegetables and fruit. You may drink herbal, non-caffeinated teas (Great to drink two to four cups throughout your juicing days) and pure water (You may find that you need only six cups, than your normal eight cups/day).

WHAT do I juice?

You can juice almost anything you can eat raw. Vegetables are best, especially carrots, cucumbers, beets, tomatoes, zucchini squash, romaine lettuce, sprouts, celery and cabbage. You may juice fruits along with your vegetables. Make sure that you juice more vegetables than fruit each time. Vegetables that DO NOT juice well include potatoes, eggplant, bananas and avocado.

HOW much juice to drink?

Drinking three—four 16 to 20 ounce cups/day is average, but you can have up to a gallon of juice/day.

What if I have to go to work?

Put your juice in a thermos or tightly sealed juice jar and keep it refrigerated or in a cooler tote bag.

What are the benefits of juicing?

- Mental clarity is improved and brain fog is lifted
- Rapid, safe weight loss is achieved without flabbiness
- The nervous system is balanced
- You will feel increased energy and sensory perception. The longer the fast, the bigger increase in energy and vitality. You normally need less sleep.
- Organs are revitalized
- Cellular biochemistry is harmonized
- The skin becomes silky, soft, and sensitive.
- There is greater ease of movement.
- Breathing becomes fuller, freer and deeper.
- Reduced allergy symptoms
- You can overcome addictions.
- You can stop overeating.
- The digestive system is rejuvenated and becomes more effective; the peristaltic action of the intestines (the cause of a natural bowel movement) is stronger after fasting.
- Fasting retrains your sense of taste back to more healthy food as acute sensitivity is restored.
- Fasting can increase confidence in our ability to have control over our lives and our appetite, and that our bodies are self-regulating and self-healing organisms capable of establishing balance when given the possibility to do so.
- Normal metabolic and cell oxygenation are restored.
- Detoxification—as soon as the body realizes that it's fasting it will begin to eliminate those things that cause disease, such as fat cells, arterial cholesterol plaques, mucus, tumors, stored up worries and emotions.

- Longer juice fasts enable the body to cleanse toxins that have been accumulating in your cellular tissues from birth.

How Long Should I Fast?

The length of juice fasting can range anywhere from one to 40 days. Three days is an excellent tune up. Five-day fasts are long enough to begin the process of healing and rebuilding the immune system. Ten-day fasts act as prevention to fight off illness including degenerative diseases. Twenty-one to 30 days is the standard therapy used by health sanitariums in Europe. If you deal with compulsive eating, start with shorter fasts so you may learn how to break the fast correctly. Most severe health conditions require fasts over 20 days, as it takes that long to repair damaged tissue.

You can test different ones and you will end up with a preference. I must admit that I saw a man being interviewed a long time ago who looked AMAZING for his age and he claimed to have done periodic juice fasts for several years.

How often should I fast?

The following are the most common time periods, however choose the one that you prefer:

- The first day of every week
- Once a month
- Once every season
- Once a year

Are there any fasting side effects?

There are numerous minor discomforts you may notice during juice fasting. These include:

- Feeling cold
- Light headedness/dizziness
- Bad breath

- Body odor
- Fatigue for first few days
- Constipation or diarrhea
- Stomach ache
- Acne or other skin eruptions
- Increased dreaming
- Changes in sleep patterns
- Aches and pains
- Frequent urination
- Coated tongue—a result of your body shedding toxins and cleansing itself
- Headaches—possibly the result of withdrawal from caffeine or a withdrawal in salt or sugar consumption.

What Can I Read For Support?

My first and favorite book on juice fasting was *Toxic Relief* and *Fasting Made Easy*, both by Don Colbert, M.D.

My favorite online resource is Fasting.com by Tom Coghill, who also wrote a book by the same name

Many juicing recipes are available online, or in books.

Post-fasting: the most important part!

After the fasting period, a lot of people go on the wrong diet—and waste the whole fast. DO NOT binge or eat junk foods after your fast. What you do after the juice fast is the MOST important part. Remember that after fasting you must always improve your diet! You want to only consume fresh vegetables, fruit and vegetable soup for three to seven days after extended juice fasts. I have eating plans available in a menu style journal that is a beneficial tool to use when you end your juice fast. It can help you with accountability and give you an exact plan to keep your results and your health. *(Diabetics and persons on medication requiring meals should check with their physician, of course. Fasting is not for children, pregnant women or nursing women. If there is a medical reason why you should not fast, then don't. Check with your doctor first.)*

Smoothies

What is the main difference between smoothies and juicing?

SMOOTHIES = ADDED FIBER = IMPROVED ELIMINATION

JUICING = MINIMIZED FIBER which = VACATION FOR DIGESTIVE SYSTEM because it requires next to no digestion. The nutrients are absorbed and assimilated immediately into the bloodstream.

Smoothies will:

- Save you money and time
- Ensure you are properly hydrated at the beginning of the day, something soda and coffee won't do.
- Provide you with the full spectrum of nature's bioavailable vitamins, nutrients, and antioxidants
- Give you plenty of natural fiber to ensure excellent digestion
- Provide you with the scientifically proven best "brain fuel" in the form of fructose
- Help empower your immune system
- Provide high quality carbohydrates from all the extra fruits, which give the average person a dramatic increase in energy.
- Taste great!
- Help reduce cravings
- Help provide muscle recovery and relieve soreness after a workout
- Be very low in calories and contain no cholesterol and sodium
- Help the mind and spirit experience positive transformations
- Stabilize your blood sugar and encourage your body to lose weight
- Be absorbed easily by the body by acting to pre-digest the fruits and vegetables (a blender is a perfect set of teeth) for better digestion. It is true that most of us do not chew our foods long enough.

Green Smoothies: What are they?

It's quite simple really. Green smoothies are smoothies with greens blended through them. Brought to the masses by raw food pioneer, chef, author and educator Victoria Boutenko, the green smoothie is a nutritional powerhouse! Greens are incredibly nutritious, however people struggle to eat enough of them with regard to quantity and many find them hard to digest. It has been suggested that this is due to not having enough stomach acid or jaw strength to chew them till they are a creamy consistency. Blended greens have their structure ripped apart and are effectively pre-digested. Adding fruit makes them taste great and is also a clever way of getting a lot of fruit into your diet, which most people don't have enough of in addition to getting your daily dose of greens.

According to Ms. Boutenko, greens are the primary food group that matches human nutritional needs most completely. Greens are loaded with amino acids, (the building blocks of protein), minerals, vitamins, fiber & chlorophyll. Greens can be combined with any other food and enhance digestion by stimulating enzyme production. Hence the combination of greens and fruit in green smoothies is very acceptable i.e. versus the combination of fruit with other food types, and starch with protein e.g. classic SAD fair such as cheese and bread, milk and cereal, etc.

What does it do? (You will notice the following to the MAX!)

More energy

- Less body aches and pain
- Normalized blood sugar
- Reduced or "cured" insomnia
- Increased libido
- Clearer thought
- Better vision

- Regular digestion
- Regular bowel movements
- Less acne
- Radiant skin
- Less illness
- Increased fiber intake
- Easy weight loss
- Increased consumption of fruits and vegetables (particularly greens)
- Fewer mood swings
- Hair and nails grow in faster and stronger
- You may feel an urge to start exercising
- Reduced craving for coffee, caffeinated drinks and sweets

. . . and the positive benefits go on . . . .

How do you make them?

The best green smoothie recipe is the one you make yourself. It's very easy and the options are endless. Just have a ration of about 50% fruits and 50% vegetables (or try some wild greens such as nettles) and your smoothie will always be delicious. Although they are green, you will be shocked at how yummy it tastes. You'll barely taste the vegetables, if at all. (And they're a great way to get vegetables into your kids!)

How Much Do I drink? 1—2 quarts (A half to 1½ blender full)

TIPS:
~Although you can add anything from simple to exotic fruits, some offer so many benefits you'll want to use them often. Ex: Blueberries are one of nature's most powerful antioxidants and their benefits are numerous. Keep your smoothies simple and do not add 12 fruits into one smoothie.

~You want to mainly use fresh fruit and add in a few pieces of out of season frozen fruit. The good news on frozen fruit is it was picked at peak times and then frozen. The bad news is that typically it is blanched (cooked for a short time) before frozen.

~Add any liquid, powder or seed supplements to your smoothie for even more of a powerful boost.

~Add water, ice and fruit. Eliminate the habit of adding milk, yogurt or juice (unless it's fresh squeezed juice).

~Remember, you are drinking calories so consider them. Some people think drinks are different.

~Drink your smoothie alone without eating anything else at that time. Not even a bite of toast!

Best Blenders:

Low to mid priced blenders: Sunbeam, Hamilton Beach and Cuisinart

Mid to high priced blenders: Vitamix, Blendtec and Waring

Fitness is my 2nd pillar in my 4-pillar system. Our bodies are made to move and fitness was never originally designed just for an aesthetic purpose. Our bodies need it to operate and function to the highest degree. Fitness/exercise is not optional but absolutely necessary. So let's discuss specifically why & how.

CHAPTER 8

R U Ready to get down & dirty?

Exercise

When you engage in physical activity, you burn calories. The more intense the activity, the more calories you burn—and the easier it is to keep your weight under control. The reason I decided to specialize specifically in boot camp-style fitness training is because I believe it is the most comprehensive and successful workout for achieving your desired body in the fastest and most varied way possible. Fitness boot camps are intense exercise sessions that challenge every muscle in your body. By rapidly moving from exercise to exercise with little rest in between, you tone and firm muscles while getting a good cardiovascular workout at the same time. Building muscle is essential to boosting the body's metabolism as well as effectively and efficiently losing weight by burning more calories throughout the day.

Fitness boot camp consists of lots of (HIIT) High Intensity Interval Training. HIIT is cardio performed at such an intense level that your body will spend the rest of the day expending energy to recover from the rigorous training you gave it. This is commonly referred to as EPOC (excess post-exercise oxygen consumption) and it means that you consume a great deal more oxygen recovering from the exercise bout than you would have if you'd just done a steady-state workout. You will be burning up to nine times more fat while sitting on the couch later that night than you would have if you'd spent an hour on the treadmill at a moderate pace. This type of training is far superior to steady-state exercises when it comes to increasing your VO2 max, which is the maximum amount of oxygen you can uptake during exercise.

Boot camp classes are a great way to alleviate boredom found in your regular routine. You know the same one you've been doing for the last year and haven't seen any results. Best of all, boot camp workouts are usually performed outdoors so it will get you out of the gym and into a new, fresh, natural environment. Fresh air cleans our lungs & exercises performed outdoors in fresh air offer increased aerobic benefits. More clean air in helps to improve our breathing technique. Better technique increases stamina. More oxygen to the muscles reduces that lactic acid build-up in the muscles which leads to cramping.

Fitness boot camps allow you to interact with others, building *camaraderie* and promoting a sustained commitment to fitness. Participants seem to support one another and reach new fitness levels together. They also inspire one another by their progress on the field, their new clothing sizes or their success in making a lifestyle change with their diet. I see strangers become friends in each boot camp as well as beginners who initially felt intimidated feeling extremely motivated by others.

Overall Benefits of Exercise

- Reduces some of the effects of aging
- Contributes to your mental well-being and helps treat depression
- Helps relieve stress and anxiety
- Increases your energy and endurance
- Helps you sleep better
- Helps you maintain a normal weight by increasing your metabolism (the rate you burn calories)
- Improves your chances of living longer

- Improves quality of life
- Reduces the risk of heart disease
- Helps lower high blood pressure (hypertension) and high cholesterol
- Helps protect you from developing certain cancers
- Helps prevent or control type 2 diabetes (adult-onset diabetes)
- Reduces the risk of arthritis and alleviates associated symptoms
- Helps prevent osteoporosis (gradual loss of bone mass/ strength)
- Improves mobility and strength in later life
- Alleviates symptoms of depression and anxiety
- Gives you a break from your daily activities and worries

Benefits of Aerobic Exercise

- Increased maximal oxygen consumption (VO_2max)
- Improvement in cardiovascular/cardiorespiratory function (heart and lungs)
- Increased maximal cardiac output (amount of blood pumped every minute)
- Increased maximal stroke volume (amount of blood pumped with each beat)
- Increased blood volume and ability to carry oxygen
- Reduced workload on the heart (myocardial oxygen consumption) for any given submaximal exercise intensity
- Decreases insulin requirement
- Increases glycogen storage
- Better hunger control
- Increased blood supply to muscles and ability to use oxygen
- Lower heart rate and blood pressure at any level of submaximal exercise
- Increased threshold for lactic acid accumulation
- Lower resting systolic and diastolic blood pressure in people with high blood pressure

- Increased HDL Cholesterol (the good cholesterol)
- Decreased blood triglycerides
- Reduced body fat and improved weight control

Benefits of Strength Training

- Increased muscular strength
- Increased strength of tendons and ligaments
- Potentially improves flexibility
- Better performance of everyday activities
- Reduced body fat and increased lean body mass
- Increased muscle strength, power, and endurance
- Potentially decreases resting systolic and diastolic blood pressure
- Positive changes in blood cholesterol
- Muscle helps you burn additional calories
- Aids rehabilitation and recovery—One of the best ways to heal many types of injuries is to strengthen muscles surrounding the injured area. The stronger your muscles, the quicker the healing process.
- Improved glucose tolerance and insulin sensitivity
- Improved strength, balance, and functional ability in older adults
- Improved balance, flexibility, mobility and stability
- Heart disease risk is lower when the body is leaner
- Improved posture because of strengthening the neck, shoulder, back, hip and abdominal muscles

Top 12 Fitness Mistakes

1. Working out a just a little bit. This may seem too obvious to belong here, but a lot of people lift two dumbbells a couple of times and think they're done for the day. Sit down at the table for half an hour and come up with a sound training program. Keep in mind

that most people do not push themselves with intensity or variety daily, so know yourself. If you don't know enough to make your own program, then work with a certified personal trainer.

2. Thinking that working out 50 hours a day is the key. Muscles need time to grow and the body needs time to burn fat. Some people think that the body only burns fat during exercises, but this is not true. The more muscles mass you have, the faster calories get burnt because muscles need energy for maintenance all the time; even when you're resting. Overtraining will simply make you tired without any additional benefits.

3. Believing you can eat anything if you exercise. All the exercise or gadgets in the world won't help you lose weight, get in shape, or live healthier if you don't follow a healthy eating plan. What all the infomercials fail to tell you is that all of those hard-body models using their equipment also tailor their diet to get them to their goals.

4. Comparing yourself to others. We are all unique individuals with unique histories of eating and fitness levels. You shouldn't rate your performance according to the achievements of others, but stick to your own goals and focus on your own success.

5. Not stretching before or after workouts. Stretching seems to be a 'lost art,' but it can improve range of motion and flexibility, and reduce the risk of muscle tightness and strain.

6. The all or nothing approach. Ever skip a whole workout because you didn't have a full hour to spare? Use what time you do have. If your goal is to wait for the perfect month to start working out or eating healthy, . . . good luck with that . . . let me know how that works out for you.

7. Doing the same things over and over. There's no better way to lose motivation than doing the same exercises in the same order over and over again. Learn to juggle around with the exercises that form your routine and replace them with new ones frequently. Find variations on a classic exercise and try them out. Make things interesting for yourself.

8. Alcoholic beverages have extra calories that you don't want. They are also metabolized as fat and very quickly. Pumping iron in the gym for 45 minutes and then throwing the entire effort away with a couple of beers is not a good way to move forward.

9. Thinking cardio is enough and skipping strength training exercises. True rehabilitation and long-term improvements only come by strengthening your muscles. Strength training does not necessarily mean "body building," but increasing muscle strength and stability.

10. Losing focus instead of practicing mindful exercise and thinking about the muscles you're working until you can feel the resistance in those areas. Concentrate on the reason you are performing each exercise. This focus will help you get more out of your workouts in less time, while assuring you use proper biomechanics. This is also why gymgoers should not be watching TV or reading magazines while working out.

11. Thinking that starvation is the key. This is a huge mistake and a lot of people do it. Never assume that you can tank your way through a fitness program while starving yourself because you'll only end up in a hospital. Muscles need nourishing meals in order to grow and starvation is a bad way to diet anyway.

12. And, lastly, never look for a magic fix that can save you all the trouble. You can't lose weight sitting around and moping in front of the TV or computer. It just doesn't happen. Some people say, "I can't do a boot camp or a raw detox because that requires work and commitment." Unfortunately some people put their hope in things that require nothing and they get nothing. So get out and take some action TODAY. And no excuses!

CHAPTER 9

R U Ready to change your mind?

Mindset is the 4ᵗʰ pillar in my 4-pillar system, but it is the most important. Because if you do not have the right mindset you will not take the necessary actions to follow through and continue with the other 3 pillars. Let's dig a little deeper in the mind and anytime it comes up throughout this book play close attention.

Detox and The Mind

Many clients have asked me if it is normal to have negative emotions arise during a juice fast or a raw detox. The answer is a resounding YES! You are surely detoxing the mind as well as the body. The following excerpt from the book, *Eating in Freedom* by Tom McGregor describes it perfectly.

> "Emotions and thinking are affected; old memories and negative feelings arise from the dead, like a detox of the soul. It is easy to become discouraged, feel irritated, short-tempered or mildly depressed. These cleansing periods require faith that it will pass. Energy packets of glycogen are stored in the liver and muscles for use during bursts of physical activity.
>
> During The Downs and Dips, the body utilizes glycogen from the liver and muscles for energy. This results in the familiar feeling of weakness. During a peak, the body has an abundant

supply of glucose, and glycogen replacement occurs at a rapid rate creating abundant energy. Also, there is an intermediate state when glycogen is starting to be replaced. You will feel energetic but lack the endurance to match. Persevering through these various fasting states and energy levels is necessary for success."

A client once told me that during her 30-day detox, feelings of an unresolved family issue came up that caused her to feel extremely emotional and she was prompted to call her sister. The sister confided that she had been thinking on the same situation lately. They ended up crying together and truly releasing the situation, creating a stronger bond with one another.

Our Best Body Part: The Brain

I really like an online hair-care forum and visit it because I get great tips and learn about products, techniques, members' trials and errors and get to see many pictures for inspiration. Many of the girls, myself included, seem to be really "into" their hair, so I posed a question to find out if they are really "into" their health/fitness. I said, "You love your hair so I know you're not fat." Some people were offended and some were curious as to where I was going with that question. Many people mentioned that it is easy and fun to focus on hair (they felt that you can quickly see results), but that with fitness/eating, they can't seem to find the motivation. I also heard many excuses as to why they can't or choose not to work out or eat healthy.

What I want to do now is show you how you can take your passion or interest for one thing (ie. hair, shopping, earning a degree etc.) and use it to have success in any area of your life, particularly health and fitness.

Four Parts of the Brain

Left Brain (words, logic)—Focuses on reality, focuses on details, reading, writing

Right Brain (patterns, images)—Focuses on changing reality, the broad picture, creative imaging

Mid-Brain (emotions)

Brain Stem (physical stimulation)—Most of us go through our days on auto-pilot, not thinking about our goals and how to obtain them. A big step in realizing your fitness/eating goals is to make it a PRIORITY, not just when you "feel like it". I will never forget this example: If a serial killer is plotting to kill someone, he has tacked on the walls details of their location, pictures, some of their belongings etc. Because of his focus he can get his target. He is not out at a party somewhere dancing and then says, "Oh man I am supposed to be killing someone right now."

The next thing to remember is that you have to use ALL four parts of the brain to hit your goals quickly and effortlessly. When one or more parts are left out, (as most people tend to do), reaching goals becomes that much harder. It takes the sum of all the parts to get it right.

The last thing to remember is to counteract negative thoughts, excuses and self-sabotage by repeating your affirmation with a feeling of joy.

Here are the actions you have to take now:

1. Write a one—or two—sentence written objective and underline it. This is your affirmation. An example is "I easily attain my fitness goals from working out 5x/wk and eating healthy. I enjoy the process and know that it is the best way for me and everyone involved."

2. Give your goal a name, so it comes to memory more easily. Ex. "Operation Fit Plan"

3. Use as many senses as possible when thinking of your Operation Fit Plan and experience total joy, success and excitement.

4. Look at your written affirmation, say it and feel it several times per day. Your brain will give you several objections/complaints during the course of a day, and by speaking your affirmation you give it life as well as build the resolve to make it happen.

Correlation between loving hair and loving to be fit:

Left-Brain (words, logic)

Hair:	Read comments in hair forums; participate, which is like saying/speaking
Fitness/Eating:	Reading and saying affirmation, reading books, belonging to fit/eating online community.

Right-Brain (patterns, images)

Hair:	Seeing before and after pictures or seeing pics of inspirational hairstyles
Fitness/Eating:	Seeing before and after pics or pics of inspirational bodies

Mid-Brain (emotions)

Hair:	Excited by the possibilities
Fitness/Eating:	Excited by the possibilities

Brain Stem (physical stimulation)

Hair:	Physically doing your hair
Fitness/Eating:	Physically working out, grocery shopping for healthy foods, preparing and eating them

More on the Power of Words

Words create impressions, images and expectations. They build psychological connections. They influence how we think. Since thoughts determine actions, there's a powerful connection between the words we use and the results we get.

The Bible teaches that words, especially ones *you* say, are important.

A man's stomach shall be satisfied from the fruit of his mouth, and from the produce of his lips he shall be filled. Death and life are in the power of the tongue, and those who love it will eat its fruit. (Proverbs 18:20-21 NKJV)

All success books teach on the power in speaking what you desire. I have been doing this for many years. I can definitely say that I get what I say ALWAYS! These are my own personal health/fitness affirmations that I say every day. It makes it easy and fun to do the things necessary to stay fit and healthy.

1. I am whole, perfect, loving, healthy, happy and harmonious.
2. I am passionate about the fitness and health of myself and others.
3. I eat and crave mostly organic fruit and vegetables.
4. My body is emotionally and physically cleansed.
5. It is very easy for me to live a healthy lifestyle.
6. It is very easy for me to stay at my desired size.
7. Being disciplined and committed to health/fitness spills over into other areas of my life.

~Always put your affirmations in present tense and never speak the negative, i.e. instead of saying "I will never eat junk anymore," say, "I only crave healthy, nutritious meals and snacks."

~It is ok if you don't believe what you say at first. The more you say it, the more it will become ingrained in your subconscious and become your reality.

~Seven is the number of completion.

More on the Power of Visualization

Many studies have been conducted that show when athletes visualize their plays and wins, they get more plays and wins. In the 1920s, followers of Freudian psychology also preached the benefits of visualization, but for different reasons. They believed that visualizing the future influences the unconscious mind, and in turn, the psychological dynamics of the unconscious would push you toward what you visualized, without your even realizing it. Again, the fundamental philosophy of self-improvement at work is that psychology is destiny, and visualizing the future is crucial for motivation and success.

==> Why Visualization Really Works

Recent sports psychology research has made it clear that visualization can enhance success and performance in sports. But parallel research in positive psychology has confirmed that visualization can enhance success in everyday life, making it a valuable tool for those interested in motivation, self-help, and self-improvement. But the reasons that visualization enhances the psychology of success are more practical and pragmatic than followers of Freudian psychology or popular self-help movements would have us believe. Here are the three main reasons that visualization enhances success and self-improvement:

1) Visualization enhances confidence

Research in the field of positive psychology shows that simply thinking about an event makes it seem more likely that it will actually happen. As you think about an event, you begin to construct mental scenarios of how it might occur, and even more importantly, how you might *make* it happen. The result is often greater confidence, and self-improvement occurs via a "self-fulfilling prophecy." The psychological process is simple:

Visualization => Confidence ==> Action ==> Results ==> Success

2) Visualization boosts motivation

Visualization boosts motivation as well as confidence, making self-help and self-improvement more effective. As your dreams for the future seem more likely, you become more motivated to initiate and sustain action.

Setting goals is often a very rational, even "dry" element of one's efforts for self-improvement. But visualizing your desired future is a very different psychological process, making abstract goals very tangible and concrete in your mind. This process engages your emotions as well as your thoughts, and generates an authentic excitement that motivates self-improvement.

Visualizing your future also makes you aware of the gap between where you are now, and where you want to be. The result is more motivation for self-improvement, as you strive to close the gap between your future ambitions and your current reality.

3) Visualizing is a form of practice

This is the most important reason that visualization enhances success, but the one most often overlooked in self-help and self-improvement books. Like any kind of practice, visualizing a behavior makes you more skilled and successful when it comes time to actually engage in that behavior. Moreover, visualized behaviors can be practiced more quickly, easily, and frequently than actual behavior—that's part of why world-class athletes regularly complement their actual practice sessions with regimens of psychologically-focused visualized practice.

Visualization is also used routinely in psychology and self-improvement because it is excellent for practicing behaviors that are too frightening, intimidating, or even dangerous to perform in person. For example . . .

If you magnify your images of your new body walking confidently down the street, you minimize the thought of deprivation of high fat/salt/sugar foods. Psychotherapists routinely ask patients to visualize themselves facing their fears and anxieties as a way of easing them into actually confronting those fears.

You can use these techniques to accomplish your fitness and eating goals!

More on Pictures

To test if encouraging people to photograph everything they ate might also encourage them to change their diet, scientists from the

University of Wisconsin-Madison asked 43 people to record what they ate for one week in pictures as well as in words. Researchers who carried out the study found that people began to eat healthier food when they were asked to take a picture of what they were eating. They believe that the pictures appear to have concentrated the dieter's mind at just the right time, before they were about to eat. The photographs were also more effective at encouraging volunteers to watch what they ate than traditional written food diaries.

When the volunteers were later quizzed, the photo diary appeared more effective at encouraging them to change their eating habits to more healthy alternatives. The photographs also acted as a powerful reminder of any snacking binges, the researchers found. "I had to think more carefully about what I was going to eat because I had to take a picture of it," was a typical response from volunteers.

I encourage my clients to take a picture of their meals and put it on my membership site, *R3Fitworld.com*. It gives that component of accountability and also allows people to share recipe ideas or just feel confirmed that others are participating in this health journey as well. With today's social media, mobile phone and uploading technology, you can jump in and start noticing the benefits.

The Start of Something New

Many people start something new in their health/fitness endeavors on January 1st. It will be my honor to help you stay on target so that it is not short lived, regardless of when you decide to start. But first, let's find out why the beginning of something is always the hardest. We are creatures of habit and fear jumps in to try and prevent us from starting new things. Here are some things that we have usually been afraid or apprehensive about starting throughout our lives:

- A new school
- A new relationship

- A new career
- A new location
- Giving birth for the first time

Let's elaborate on the first birth . . . . you do not know what to expect, except that there is pain (because that is what you've been told). You want to think of the end result only but for some reason you focus instead on the pain and discomfort. You don't know exactly how long it will take so you grow impatient. Friends and family have told you their experiences, but you feel overwhelmed and just want it to be over now! You start to question yourself and wonder if you can actually deliver this baby. You are starting to let the fear turn into anger. You are now on a mission and DETERMINED to push and push HARD. Your focus has changed and you want to get to the benefits. You did the morning sickness, mood swings, weight changes and discomforts but now you are ready. You give one final push and now you hear the sounds of victory. You hold this wonderful joy in your arms and KNOW that it was soooooo worth it and can't believe that you had thoughts of giving up. Now you will live out your life maintaining and encouraging the best for your bundle of joy.

Attaining and maintaining your best body encompasses the SAME patterns!

Junk Foods and the Power of Advertising

What is the purpose of food? To give us fuel, energy and life. What is the purpose of junk food? It has none, while actually diminishing energy and life. Michael S. Lasky, author of *The Complete Junk Food Book*, has this to say about eating junk food and the power of advertising:

> "We are all proselytized at an important age into consuming puppets of the junk food barons. Our parents inadvertently

help them by buying their products as a form of 'reward' food. We grow up unaware that we have slowly acquired a junk food habit by the subtle forces of advertising. By the time we are capable of making a decision about junk food, we are already hooked from years and years of indulging in what we had been told by TV was good food."

This is what Natural Hygienist Mike Benton had to say on the topic:

"Actually, very little "good food" is advertised. Eighty percent of all food advertising is for blatant junk foods. Most of the remaining 20% is for convenience foods that are often little better than the candy, cakes, and snack foods which make up the majority of food advertising. In fact, out of the top 100 most heavily advertised food products, over 30 of them have absolutely zero food value, except for empty calories."

The majority of Americans receive almost all of their nutritional information from advertising. In other words, the typical person only knows as much about nutrition and good food as the advertisers want to tell him. When asked how good a job food manufacturers do in telling the public about good nutrition, a leading advertising executive for a convenience food company said: "The job of product advertising is to persuade and sell, not to educate." Studies have shown that it does not matter how nutritious a food may be or even how good it tastes. It is advertising alone that sells a food product, and it is primarily the junk foods and the nonfoods that are advertised the heaviest.

This reminds me of a personal situation where, since I was seven years old, I had received chemical strengtheners (relaxers) on my hair. I didn't even realize the damage I was doing with exposure to these chemicals. I never questioned it because it was common for my culture and environment. Only until I happened upon a book in the library in my late 20's that showed an example of what my natural hair would look like, did I even question this disastrous routine. After reading one book I grabbed the scissors and cut all of my relaxed hair off, leaving only about an inch of my un-relaxed hair. I continued to educate myself more on my hair and natural products that would make my hair healthy. The more I got to know 'my hair', the more I loved it and the more I was outraged that I took so long to be responsible enough to learn and act on the truth. I had been living a lie on what people and advertisers were saying was best for me. Ever since that enlightening moment in the library I have been growing and taking good care of my naturally curly hair. I want you to ask yourself why you would make a choice to eat junk foods and if they "serve you" or "slave you"?

3 E's (Your Experience, Experiment and Enlightenment)

I like for my clients to use the 3 E's to test for themselves the power of the R3 eating plan.

Experience: You have your 20, 30, 40, 50 or 60+ years of eating foods. You are aware that what you have been doing makes you feel a certain way, sleep a certain way and react a certain way. You know how it has affected your health, digestion, elimination, aging, complexion, mood, weight and energy. You know which foods you are compulsive over and which ones are your 'comfort foods'. The good news is that all this information will come in handy as you test it against your new eating plan and the new benefits you experience.

Experiment: Experiment by definition is *(noun) a test, trial or tentative procedure; an act or operation for the purpose of discovering something unknown or of testing a principle, supposition*, etc. *(verb) to try or test, esp. in order to discover or prove something.* When a person or expert tries to encourage you to change for the supposed better, it is not yours yet; you do not own it! However when you test something and see all the benefits first hand, you are relieved and anxious and will start to move into the realm of enlightenment.

Enlightenment: You can now be self-motivated to continue with your new actions because they have been proven to be real in your life. You are no longer testing a theory, but gladly living it and in many cases wish you would have known sooner. I would encourage you to not get too cocky and confident now because it still has to form into a habit through repetition. You have more years of doing it the old way than the new way. Until it becomes a habit, your subconscious may try and deter you with one of your trigger foods, place or times. This is where it is beneficial to reference the mindset section to work on making this part of your healthy lifestyle for a lifetime.

CHAPTER 10

R U Ready to grocery shop & store?

Suggested Foods for Shopping

Fresh Fruit:

Apples, Apricots, Avocados, Bananas, Berries, Blueberries, Cantaloupes, Casaba Melon, Cherries, Coconuts, Cranberries, Crenshaw Melon, Durian, Figs, Grapefruits, Grapes, Honeydew Melon, Kiwi, Kumquats, Lemons, Limes, Lychees, Mangos, Mangosteen, Melons, Mulberries, Nectarines, Oranges, Papayas, Passion fruit, Peaches, Pears, Pineapples, Plums, Prunes, Raisins, Strawberries, Watermelon

Fresh Vegetables:

Alfalfa, Sprouts, Artichokes, Arugula, Asparagus, Beets, Bean Sprouts, Bok Choy, Broccoli, Brussels Sprouts, Cabbages, Carrots, Cauliflower, Celery, Chives, Collards, Corn, Cucumbers, Dandelion Greens, Eggplant, Endive, Escarole, Garlic, Green Peas, Kale, Kohlrabi, Leeks, Lettuce, Malva, Mustard Greens, Okra, Onions, Oyster Plant, Parsnips, Peppers, Potatoes, Potatoes-sweet, Radishes, Shallots, Spinach, Sprouts, String Beans, Squash, Swiss Chard, Tomatoes, Turnips, Turnip Greens, Watercress, Wheat Grass, Yams

Raw, Unsalted Nuts & Seeds
Almonds, Brazil Nuts, Cashew Nuts, Chestnuts, Filberts, Hazel Nuts, Hemp Seeds, Hulled Macadamias, Peanuts, Pecans, Pine Nuts, Pumpkin Seeds, Sesame Seeds, Sunflower Seeds, Walnuts

Nut Butters: Pumpkin Seed Butter, Almond Butter, Sesame Tahini, Macadamia Nut Butter

Natural Oils

(Cold-pressed or expeller-pressed are the best)
Almond Oil, Avocado Oil, Extra-virgin Coconut Oil, Extra-virgin Olive Oil, Flaxseed Oil, Hempseed Oil, Macadamia Oil, Safflower Oil, Sesame Seed Oil, Sunflower Oil, Walnut Oil

Beans & Legumes
Adzuki, Black, Dried, Peas, Garbanzo, Great Northern, Kidney, Lentils, Lima, Miso, Navy, Pinto, Soy, Tempeh, Tofu

Natural Organic Whole Grains
Amaranth, Barley, Basmati, White Rice, Brown Rice, Buckwheat, Bulgur Wheat, Corn Meal, Couscous, Flax, Millet, Oats, Pasta, Quinoa, Rye, Wheat, Wild Rice

Seafood
Char, Clams, Crab, Cod, Flounder, Halibut, Herring, Mackerel, Sablefish, Salmon, Sardines, Scallops, Shrimp, Squid, Tilapia, Trout, Tuna

Organic Grass Fed, Free-Range Poultry/ Meats
Beef, Chicken, Lamb, Turkey, Venison

Spices/Herbs
Basil, Black Pepper, Chili Pepper, Cilantro, Coriander, Cloves, Cumin, Dill, Fenugreek, Ginger Seeds, Lemongrass, Marjoram, Mint, Mustard, Oregano, Parsley, Rosemary, Saffron, Sage, Thyme, Turmeric

Top 15 Fruits to Buy Organic

Apples, Apricots, Bananas, Cherries, Grapes, Honeydew Melons, Kiwi, Lemons, Limes, Nectarines, Oranges, Peaches, Pears, Raspberries, Strawberries

Top 15 Vegetables to Buy Organic

Bell Peppers, Carrots, Cauliflower, Celery, Corn, Cucumbers, Green Beans, Hot Peppers, Kale, Leafy Greens, Potatoes, Tomatoes, Winter Squash, (whole-grain) Oats, (whole –grain) Rice

Storage Location: Fruits, Melons, Vegetables

- Store garlic, onions, potatoes, and sweet potatoes in a well-ventilated area in the pantry. Protect potatoes from light to avoid greening.

Store in refrigerator:

Fruits
- Apples (more than seven days)
- Apricots
- Blackberries
- Blueberries
- Cherries
- Cut fruits
- Figs
- Grapes
- Nashi (Asian pears)
- Raspberries
- Strawberries

Vegetables
- Artichokes
- Asparagus
- Green beans
- Lima beans

- Beets
- Belgian endive
- Broccoli
- Brussels sprouts
- Cabbage
- Carrots
- Cauliflower
- Celery
- Cut vegetables
- Green onions
- Herbs (not basil)
- Leafy vegetables
- Leeks
- Lettuce
- Mushrooms
- Peas
- Radishes
- Spinach
- Sprouts
- Summer squashes
- Sweet corn

Ripen on the counter first, then store in the refrigerator:
- Avocados
- Kiwi fruit
- Nectarines
- Peaches
- Pears
- Plums
- Pluots

Store only at room temperature:
- Apples (fewer than seven days)
- Bananas

- Basil (in water)
- Cucumbers†
- Dry onions*
- Eggplant†
- Garlic*
- Ginger
- Grapefruit
- Jicama
- Lemons
- Limes
- Mandarins
- Mangoes
- Muskmelons
- Oranges
- Papayas
- Peppers†
- Persimmons
- Pineapple
- Plantains
- Pomegranates
- Potatoes*
- Pumpkins
- Sweet potatoes*
- Tomatoes
- Watermelons
- winter squashes

†Cucumbers, eggplant, and peppers can be kept in the refrigerator for one to three days if they are used soon after removal from the refrigerator.

*These should be stored in a cool, dry environment with good ventilation. Paper bags, cardboard boxes, and pantries are good places to store them. An ideal temperature for storage would be between 45 and 55 degrees Fahrenheit. Avoid storing them in plastic bags or in refrigerators and make sure the environment is not too warm.

Storage Location C or P Meals

Organize your carbohydrates and animal proteins by category. When it is time for you to have your C or P Meal, you could easily reach in and grab something from a different shelf to ensure variety.

Shopping Tips

- Shop twice per week to retain freshness and minimize spoilage.
- Shop for a colorful variety of produce to get all of the benefits they each contain.
- Shop at local farmers markets, health food stores or sign up for a (preferably organic) produce co-op to get fresh produce at great savings
- Consider growing a garden.
- Purchase free-range grass fed animal products whenever possible.
- Do not shop at more than two grocery stores. Mentally it can wear you down and it may end up costing you more in gasoline than the $1 you save on cherries.
- Do not buy any junk foods (especially in bulk sizes).

Handling fruits and vegetables

Most people do not realize the crucial importance of freshness when it comes to produce. Whenever we slice into a vegetable or fruit we expose the cut surfaces to heat, light and oxygen—the nutrient destroyers. This exposure results in the oxidation of phytonutrients and loss of some nutritional value of the fruit or vegetable. An example of oxidation can be seen by cutting an apple, pear or banana and letting it sit in the open a few minutes. The "browning" you observe is evidence of the oxidation that robs it of its nutrients. Antioxidant protection can be seen by taking the type of same fruit or vegetable and cutting it up but this time apply some "fruit fresh" crystals (a brand of produce protectors that keeps fresh cut fruit fresh for up to eight hours) and notice how the crystals prevent oxidation, which is the antioxidant protecting the fruit. Some fresh orange juice will work too. In the natural state, fruits and vegetables are provided protection from the air because of their skins. Even though they still "go bad in time," the protection of their skins is lost when they are cut up, diced or sliced.

According to Nutritional Medicine specialist Dr. Ray D. Strand, "Fresh salads and cut vegetables and fruit lose more than 40 to 50 percent of their value if they sit for more than three hours." All I know is that I incorporate tons of fruits and vegetables into my eating plan to receive their benefits. If I were not concerned about nutrients, I would just plow down pizzas and burgers and the like and call it a day. But since that is not the case, and I am going to eat premium foods, WHY would I allow nutrient depletion just so I could have the "convenience" of pre-sliced produce? A good rule of thumb is "If I cut it now, I eat it now." The only exception is if cutting them the night before will help your days run more efficiently and ensure you eat it then do so. Just make sure you seal them in an air tight container and refrigerate.

Helpful Charts

Soaking and Sprouting Times

Nut / Seed	Dry Amount	Soak Time	Sprout Time	Sprout Length	Yield
Alfalfa Seeds	3 Tbsp	12 Hours	3-5 Days	1-2 Inches	4 cups
Almonds	3 Cups	8-12 Hours	1-3 Days	1/8 Inch	4 Cups
Amaranth	1 Cup	3-5 Hours	2-3 Days	1/4 Inch	3 Cups
Barley, Hulled	1 Cup	6 Hours	12-24 Hours	1/4 Inch	2 Cups
Broccoli Seed	2 Tbsp	8 Hours	3-4 Days	1-2 Inches	2 Cups
Buckwheat, Hulled	1 Cup	6 Hours	1-2 Days	1/8-1/2 Inch	2 Cups
Cabbage Seed	1 Tbsp	4-6 Hours	4-5 Days	1-2 Inches	1 1/2 Cups
Cashews	3 Cups	2-3 Hours			4 Cups
Clovers	3 Tbsp	5 Hours	4-6 Days	1-2 Inches	4 Cups
Fenugreek	4 Tbsp	6 Hours	2-5 Days	1-2 Inches	3 Cups
Flax Seeds	1 Cup	6 Hours			2 Cups
Garbanzo Beans (Chick Pea)	1 Cup	12-48 Hours	2-4 Days	1/2-1 Inch	4 Cups
Kale Seed	4 Tbsp	4-6 Hours	4-6 Days	3/4-1 Inch	3-4 Cups
Lentil	3/4 Cup	8 Hours	2-3 Days	1/2-1 Inch	4 Cups
Millet	1 Cup	5 Hours	12 Hours	1/16 Inch	3 Cups
Mung Beans	1/3 Cup	8 Hours	4-5 Days	1/4-3 Inches	4 Cups
Mustard Seeds	3 Tbsp	5 Hours	3-5 Days	1/2-1 1/2 Inches	3 Cups
Oats, Hulled	1 Cup	8 Hours	1-2 Days	1/8 Inch	1 Cup
Onion Seed	1 Tbsp	4-6 Hours	4-5 Days	1-2 Inches	1 1/2-2 Cups
Pea	1 Cup	8 Hours	2-3 Days	1/2-1 Inch	3 Cups
Pinto Beans	1 Cup	12 Hours	3-4 Days	1/2-1 Inch	3-4 Cups
Pumpkin	1 Cup	6 Hours	1-2 Days	1/8 Inch	2 Cups
Quinoa	1 Cup	3-4 Hours	2-3 Days	1/2 Inch	3 Cups
Radish	3 Tbsp	6 Hours	3-5 Days	3/4-2 Inches	4 Cups
Rye	1 Cup	6-8 Hours	2-3 Days	1/2-3/4 Inch	3 Cups

Sesame Seed, Hulled	1 Cup	8 Hours			1 1/2 Cups
Sesame Seed, Unhulled	1 Cup	4-6 Hours	1-2 Days	1/8 Inch	1 Cup
Spelt	1 Cup	6 Hours	1-2 Days	1/4 Inch	3 Cups
Sunflower, Hulled	1 Cup	6-8 Hours	1 Day	1/4-1/2 Inch	2 Cups
Teff	1 Cup	3-4 Hours	1-2 Days	1/8 Inch	3 Cups
Walnuts	3 Cups	4 Hours			4 Cups
Wheat	1 Cup	8-10 Hours	2-3 Days	1/4-3/4 Inch	3 Cups
Wild Rice	1 Cup	12 Hours	2-3 Days	Rice Splits	3 Cups

The following food combining chart is from Alder Brooke Healing Arts and it is an excellent quick reference sheet outlining the best food combinations for optimal & efficient digestion. (Refer to pg. 15 for a more thorough explanation of food combining.)

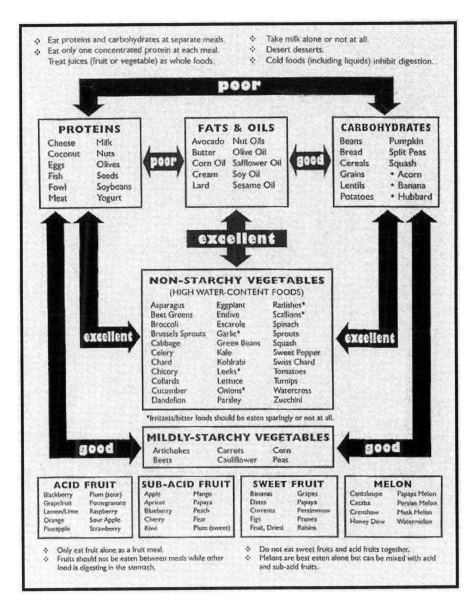

CHAPTER 11

R U Ready to hear from others?

BEWARE of people

Your main temptations will come because of family, friends, strangers or yourself. In other words, every possible problem will come from a person or people. There are many ways in which people can intentionally or unintentionally stunt your progress. It could be family questioning your eating plan that causes you to reconsider doing what's truly healthy. Friends can invite you to social parties or luncheons that cause you to want to ignore your eating plan. You can see strangers on billboards, magazines or on TV that seem to be enjoying life while eating anything at anytime, causing you to question the necessity of your eating plan. Finally, you have your own daily thoughts and temptations that can cause you to fail if you give heed to them. That is why the mindset section of this book is so important and powerful. It will give you everything you need to follow this plan happily and easily, not to mention how positively it can affect the other areas of your life.

Real Life Scenarios (the names have been changed to protect the individual's privacy (to R names of course):

Problem: Rose had been overweight since she was 16. She was raised in a poor household and her diet consisted of mainly processed foods. There was never a lot of food at home and so she had a "feast or famine" cycle of eating. When she became a young adult she ate out at drive-thru's for over half of her meals. She is now married with two kids and is considered obese. She came to us, committed to fitness and even committed to the 30-day raw detox. She lost 16 lbs and 18 inches. Unfortunately she did not commit to the *R3 Diet* after her detox. Month after month she stayed committed to fitness, but went back to her old, comfortable ways of eating. When asked why, she stated that she knew how to shop for those foods, she liked the taste and she felt they were less expensive.

Solution based on my Four Pillars:

Food: Rose needed to view food as fuel . . . premium fuel for a premium life! She attended our lecture called, "The Top 10 Benefits for a Healthy Diet". We also took her on a grocery shopping tour to realize that healthy food can be affordable. Finally, she attended our cooking classes once a week for a few months to learn how to create healthy & simple meals in less time than she thought.

Fitness: Committed

Supplements: She is only taking a multivitamin. Once she makes R3 a natural habit, she wants to attend our supplements class to learn their purposes and to get live demonstrations. She is realizing that she is the personality type that learns and retains better by a hands-on approach.

Mindset: Rose's mindset had been heavily influenced by her upbringing and environment. This is all new to her so it is imperative that she get support & accountability with like-minded people. She joined my membership site to get expert guidance along with an online social community. She is now able to relate her story with others' and no longer feel like a failure (even if she falls back to her old habits). Now instead of falling off forever, it is very short-lived and she quickly gets back on track. Mainly because the website is a reminder as to why she wants to change her lifestyle in the first place.

Problem: Rachel had struggled with weight for years and was inspired to sign up for our fitness boot camps because of popular weight-loss television shows. It was difficult for her to keep up and do many of the workouts but she did not complain and got better and stronger in time.

There was one main problem though. She was not losing much weight or inches month after month. During a consultation, I discovered that she kept doing the 30-Day raw detox for one or two weeks and then quitting. I motivated and challenged her to do the 30-day raw till completion. She finally did the full 30 days successfully, lost 20 lbs & 24 inches and was given instructions for R3. I found out months later during another consult that she never fully did R3 and that she had been looking at other diets and finding excuses not to commit.

Solution based on my Four Pillars:

Food: Rachel is like many who are taken aback when they assume that fitness is the biggest piece of the weight-loss puzzle, only to find out that food gets that coveted position. She really does not have faith in herself letting go of the unhealthy sugary and salty snacks that she loves. She ended up signing up for a three-week stay in our fitness and weight-loss retreat. She felt that she could not resist temptation on her own and wanted to surrender control. It helped her tremendously because she took everything that she learned, and found it much easier to continue what we had started once she returned home. She is also a member of R3FitWorld.com to keep abreast of new healthy recipes, restaurants, articles and videos and more.

Fitness: Committed

Supplements: Committed

Mindset: Rachel thinks and talks like a new person. She actually encouraged many people at her job to incorporate green smoothies into their diet. Everywhere she goes people are asking her how she lost so much weight and why she seems extremely more helpful, exuberant and pleasant now. She always replies, "I feel different because I think different which causes me to act different and it is turning me to a better Rachel."

Problem: Rita is a family member who moved here temporarily to work for us. We had forewarned her years prior that her body fat % was too high and gave her the R3 as her eating plan. She rejected it and argued vehemently about how she disagrees that her body fat is that high and how her lifestyle is fine the way it was. She was not open to change because she did not think it was needed and hearing it from a younger family member only made her rebel more against the idea.

Solution based on my Four Pillars:

Food: Rita started the 30-day raw detox simultaneously upon moving to town. She said that she felt better than she ever had and lost an impressive amount of weight and body fat at the end of her detox. She left town for a short time and confessed that she had felt over-confident from her results and started slowly creeping back to her old way of eating. When she came back in town and re-measured, she was thoroughly disappointed and immediately committed to the R3. At the end of her time of working with our company Rita had reached a body fat and weight that she had not seen since high school. She used to get sick frequently, including frequent headaches and now she rarely gets sick. She enjoys grocery shopping, reading health articles and enjoying healthy and tasty meals. She follows R3 easily and happily now because she has now retrained her old habits successfully.

Fitness: Committed

Supplements: Committed

Mindset: Rita had a stubborn mindset that was in denial. She overcame that by being more open minded. She did a little research on her own. She attended R3 lectures and participated on R3FitWorld. com. She appreciates and values the whole experience and can now be fit, healthy and R3 for life.

Problem: Ramiro started our program reluctantly as his wife dragged him. He did not have confidence that he could do anything we were asking of him. He was middle-aged & obese with a very large & protruding pot belly and had been sedentary for years. He was about to start fitness boot camp the next week and had just finished his first lecture on the 30-day raw detox when he approached me after class. He informed me that he was Italian and that there was NO WAY he could only eat raw fruits, vegetables & nuts for 30 days. He also informed me that he had not worked out in years and to "cut him some slack" at the fitness boot camp.

Solution based on my Four Pillars:
   Food: Ramiro was exposed to the fact that he was just making excuses and that if he really wanted help he would no longer be able to think problem-means-ruined but needed to think problem-find-solution. He ended up successfully completing the raw detox (with his wife's help) and fitness boot camp. He started R3 and shortly thereafter moved away, but still remained on R3. He sends updates to us periodically letting us know that he is looking younger than he ever has and feeling better than he ever had. He is maintaining R3 for life.
   Fitness: Committed
   Supplements: Committed
   Mindset: Ramiro's mindset had to go through the reverse, retrain, rebuild cycle like many people. He seemed opposed to trying in the beginning, but once he started seeing the benefits, he wanted more of them. His results ended up being a huge motivator for him to allow his mindset to be changed.

Problem: Roxy had been a fashion model for years. She felt that the only way for her to compete in the industry was to be as thin as possible by any means possible. She was under-nourished and under-fed but she did not know of any other way to achieve a small clothing size. She came to us in her mid-thirties. She no longer modeled and was now overweight from eating the standard American diet that consisted of high fat, high salt, high sugar and high processed foods.

Solution based on my Four Pillars:
   Food: Roxy completed the 30-day raw detox successfully and was immediately in a position to hit her dream body weight and inches in just one more boot camp. She started the *R3 Diet* and at the end of that one's month session she was at her desired weight and inches. It has

been over two years and she is still in our fitness boot camp program, and enjoying R3 for life!

Fitness: Committed

Supplements: Committed

Mindset: Roxy had very few struggles because she started our program with a VERY open & willing mindset. She acknowledged that her ways of trying to be healthy, fit and trim were NOT working and was optimistic about trying a new and proven way. She is a faithful member of R3FitWorld.com. I also later found out that she was using a "thankful journal" to record daily things for which she was thankful.

Problem: Randy has always "appeared" healthy! He looks fit. He frequently runs marathons. He's successful and happy in his career and family life. He's well traveled and smart . . . . .but he had dangerously high cholesterol levels. His body fat % was a lot higher than anyone would have imagined.

Solution based on my Four Pillars:

Food: Randy successfully completed the 30-day raw detox. His medical doctor was so impressed by his lab work and the fact that his cholesterol went from 185 from 84 in four weeks that he vowed to recommend us to more of his patients. Randy's body fat % went into a healthy range and his skin started to look even younger and more radiant. He started eating R3 for life!

Fitness: Committed

Supplements: He started learning and implementing supplements into his daily way of eating.

Mindset: Randy was busy living a full and satisfying life and never really took the time to learn how to make it more fulfilling by optimizing his health. His mindset is very positive and he enjoys reaping the rewards of his renewed health and shares his new knowledge with other friends and family.

Problem: Rhonda was one of our oldest female clients in her mid to late 60's. She second guessed herself after starting our program as she noticed she was one of the oldest participants. She also wasn't too keen on starting the 30-day raw detox, so she inquired with her medical doctor to try and get him to discourage her to do it. Finally she told me that her adult daughter suggested to her that she change from our five day/wk program to the three day/wk program because of her age.

Food: To Rhonda's surprise her doctor told her that he had been encouraging her to change her diet for the longest and that he thinks the 30-day raw would be a great jumpstart to that. She made a full commitment to the 30-day raw and said that it was difficult but doable. She said the benefits far outweighed any discomforts.

Fitness: I encouraged Rhonda to keep her five/days a week fitness regimen as the body will get acclimated faster and build endurance and strength faster on the five-day. She kept it and even showed up to boot camp when there was a horrendous thunderstorm with tornado warnings (She was the ONLY one by the way), which shows how her mindset strengthened greatly.

Supplements: Committed

Mindset: See (fitness above)

Problem: Raquel came to us as a skinny/fat/unhealthy person. She looked thin, but had a high body fat %. She looked years older than her age from years of unhealthy eating and drug and alcohol abuse. Raquel stared at me in an outraged kind of way during my 30-day raw detox lecture. After the class she asked me what seemed to be a long list of endless questions. Finally, she agreed to do it as long as she could text and email me questions during that time (We did not have the membership site at that point).

Solution based on my 4 pillars:

Food: Raquel took me up on my word and contacted me several times each week as she did the 30-day raw detox. She came to every class we offered and many classes around the community. She actually ended up making delicious gourmet raw recipes that she discovered from books, classes or online. Raquel started R3 and was successful until during one of her measurement evaluations, I noticed something was off. I found out that she started making lots of gourmet snacks and desserts and was "snacking" between meals. She eliminated the snacking, continued on with R3 and is where she should optimally be.

Fitness: Committed

Supplements: Committed

Mindset: Raquel had an inquisitive mindset. She truly wanted to understand how she could successfully start and complete the 30-day raw. After she saw the positive changes in her body and mind from the raw detox she truly wanted to know how to successfully implement the *R3 Diet*. She went into it like playing a new board game; explain the rules and tools and let me play! She currently is on R3FitWorld.com frequently and is R3 for life!

Problem: Raven was morbidly obese and considering having bariatric weight loss surgery. She felt as though she had tried everything on the planet from weight-loss pills to fitness programs without any success. She said that doctors told her that she could possibly die because of the stress on her organs caused by the enormous amount of weight. She always found herself in a destructive, repetitive cycle of binge eating and depression and was desperate for a change.

Solution based on my Four Pillars:

Food: Raven preferred to sign up for our R3 Fitness Retreat to get out of her normal environment that involved people who were facilitating her wreckful behavior. Her first sign of improvement was the gratefulness and joy she felt from being around others with a similar mindset. Her depression, however, caused her to spend most of her days alone surrounded by four walls. She easily followed our eating plan as if she were finally relieved to surrender her mind from food. We witnessed drastic results in a short amount of time from Raven mentally, emotionally and physically. She left with an immeasurable amount of confidence in herself, which caused her to successfully implement R3 for life!

Fitness: Not only did Raven commit, but she never complained and was in awe that some of the other "healthier" participants seemed to complain somewhat automatically.

Supplements: Committed

Mindset: Raven did not feel as though she had anything to lose because she felt that she was already at rock bottom. She did not want to quit and she did not see any benefits in quitting. After months on R3 and constantly seeing her weight & body fat % go down and energy & resilience go up, she is experiencing life in a way that she never even imagined. Raven's mindset is now one of expectancy . . . she expects great things.

Problem: Rosalind was a professional WNBA player. She was married and had just had her 2nd child months prior. She said that she was used to her coach giving her a detailed map on fitness, food, supplements and mindset and enforcing it in assertive ways. Now that she was in a new stage of her life, she was dealing with stored body fat, making excuses for not working out and still eating cinnamon buns, which were residual cravings left from her pregnancies. She knew how accountability had helped her in the past and wanted it to redeem her once again.

Solution based on my Four Pillars:

Food: Rosalind attended every lecture we offered. She successfully completed the 30-day raw, but did give into some chicken on one of the days, so she had to add three more days onto it. She flourished on the R3 and was surprised at how she went from having "sweets" daily because of what seemed to be irresistible urges to having sweets only on birthdays, holidays and special occasions.

Fitness: Committed . . . She said now that she has seen the difference in working out or not on her self-image, confidence, health, energy, physique & mindset . . . . she will never choose an excuse over fitness again!

Supplements: Committed

Mindset: Athletes know what is like to go for a victory. Rosalind is no different! She wants the best, finds a way to attain it and goes after it with tenaciousness!

Problem: Ruth had a gym membership she never used, walked or ran every now and then and felt that her eating was pretty good and was not interested in modifying it. She signed up for our program at the urging of some of her friends, but adamantly decided NOT to do the 30-day raw detox because she felt that everything seemed too "EXTREME"!

Solution based on my Four Pillars:

Food: Ruth said that although she left the lecture intending not to do the 30-day raw, all weekend her gut/instincts were telling her she needed to do it. At the end of her detox she came and gave me a very emotional "thank you", She also told me how it changed her in numerous ways completely and how she can't keep up with the requests for info on it from her friends and family! They are noticing her positive changes and want the same experience/results. She has now been on the R3 for months and her husband has finally decided to get on board and see what all the rave is about.

Fitness: Committed

Supplements: Committed

Mindset: Ruth realized that in order to allow new thoughts, ideas & concepts into her life, she would have to let go of old, ingrained beliefs that did not serve her to the utmost. Some people are reluctant to change, but ultimately have to make a decision to change. Ruth is now enjoying many benefits due to her changed mindset.

CHAPTER 12

R U listening to your body?

Your Body Talks But Do You Listen?

These are 'early warning signs' that could be resolved with simple changes to diet or lifestyle. Many of these nutritional deficiencies or imbalances, if left unchecked, could result in serious illness or disease.

Are you a Vegan?

If you are you may be deficient in VITAMIN B12, ZINC and IRON

Vegans who eat a **balanced diet** are unlikely to be deficient but it is essential to make sure the diet is well balanced. Vegans should be very aware of their dietary needs.

Many scientific studies comparing vegetarians with typical Western diet eaters have found that vegetarians are considerably healthier and less likely to suffer from a wide range of illnesses than meat eaters, and they tend to live longer.

What's more, there are apparently no illnesses to which vegetarians seem more prone to develop than meat eaters. Since 1898, nutritionists have been telling us, "No single factor is more important in determining the outbreak of cancer in the predisposed than high feeding. Many indications point to gluttonous consumption of meat as likely to be especially harmful." (Scientific American, December 1898).

Vegetarian diets are associated with **reduced risk** for a number of chronic diseases, including: obesity, coronary artery disease, hypertension, diabetes, mellitus, colorectal cancer, lung cancer, and kidney disease. ("Position of the American Dietetic Association: Vegetarian Diets," Journal of the American Dietetic Association, Messina, V. & Burke, K., V97 No. 11, 1997, p. 1317.) In many countries of the world—developing countries where few animal products are eaten—such diseases are virtually unknown.

A vegetarian eats food that is free from any ingredients obtained from the killing of animals. A vegan eats food free from any animal products. Because there are so many foods that vegetarians DO eat, it's easier to state which they don't eat!

What is a Vegan diet?

A vegetarian does not eat red meat (eg lamb, bacon, pork, beef), white meat or poultry (eg duck, chicken, turkey), fish or other sea creatures (eg tuna, cod, prawns, lobster) or slaughterhouse byproducts (eg animal fat, gelatin, as it is made from crushed bones, horns etc). A vegetarian may or may not eat eggs and dairy products (eg cow's milk, cheese, butter, yogurt).

Vegetarians who choose to eat dairy products and eggs are LACTO-OVO VEGETARIANS.

- Those who eat dairy products but not eggs are LACTO VEGETARIANS.
- Those who eat eggs but not dairy products are OVO VEGETARIANS.
- **Those who avoid all animal products, including all dairy products, eggs and honey are VEGANS.**
- **Those who avoid all animal products, including all dairy products, eggs and honey an only eat their fruits, vegetables & nuts in its raw form are RAW FOOD VEGANS.**

Are you forgetful?

You may have a deficiency of Vitamin B.

What is forgetfulness and how does it differ from dementia?

Loss of memory is a common symptom, particular in the elderly, but memory loss may also be associated with lack of *concentration*. Many people fear a diagnosis of *Alzheimer's disease* but many other possibilities exist, including simply the normal deterioration of memory function with *aging*. Other possibilities include the side effects of various medications and other medical conditions such as *depression*, *anxiety*, *alcohol abuse*, *drug abuse*, certain brain conditions (e.g. *stroke* or *brain tumors*) and dietary deficiency.

Nutrition and memory

Occasional memory lapses are a natural part of life at any age, and memory should not necessarily deteriorate with age unless there is also Alzheimer's disease. Most memory lapses have nothing to do with this disease, however, and with proper diet and nutrition the memory should function until well into old age.

Reasons for memory loss can include insufficient supply of necessary nutrients to the brain, high cholesterol and triglycerides, insufficient nutrients to make relevant neurotransmitters, free radical damage caused by oxidation, menopause, allergies, stress, thyroid disorders, hypoglycemia and poor circulation to the brain. Boredom and not paying attention to what needs to be remembered can also be a cause for poor memory.

To improve your memory:

- Eat a diet high in raw and lightly steamed vegetables.
- Eat brewer's yeast, brown rice, millet, wheat-germ, soybeans, nuts, seeds, legumes, and eggs.

- Eat oily fish such as mackerel, salmon, herring, sardine, pilchard at least three times per week. When not eating these, take fish oil supplements.
- Avoid sugar and anything containing sugar, white flour, white rice and all refined food.
- Avoid alcohol.

Are you over 60 years of age?

If you are, you may be deficient in VITAMINS and MINERALS, especially the B VITAMINS and HYDROCHLORIC ACID.

Myth No 1.
When I get old, I'll become senile.

Many of us view the elderly as doddering old creatures, unable to think for themselves and constantly forgetting the most mundane things. In reality, senility only strikes five percent of Americans. The other piece of good news is that some age related declines in mental functioning can be prevented or even reversed.

When scientists from Tufts University reviewed a number of studies, they discovered that vitamin deficiencies account for many of the symptoms of senility. Just as vitamins are needed for normal nervous system development in children, they are required for normal neurological functioning in adults—young and old.

For example, low folate levels in the elderly can cause forgetfulness, irritability and possibly depression. Vitamin B6, a nutrient required to make many neurotransmitters, may lead to peripheral neuropathy (a disorder of the nervous system where the limbs feel numb or tingle) if deficient. The nutrient that ensures nerves are protected with a myelin sheath, vitamin B12, can be responsible for delusions and mood disturbances when levels fall below normal.

Most of us think that nutrition must be poor before these kind of deficiencies show up. However, researchers have found that seemingly healthy, elderly subjects can still exhibit low vitamin levels. In fact, an older individual can be lacking in certain vitamins for years without any hint of a deficiency. Symptoms, mental or otherwise, may not show up immediately and even the usual blood tests employed to detect lagging nutrients are not always reliable (1).

Myth No 2: Old age means losing all my teeth.

If you're not worried about losing your mind when you're old, you might fret about losing your teeth. Periodontitis, or late stage gum disease, is the primary cause of tooth loss in adults. This condition commonly begins as gingivitis where gums turn red and begin to swell and bleed, a situation experienced by too many people. Fortunately healthy gums and avoiding false teeth are both reasonable goals.

The elderly of today are much more likely to keep their teeth than previous generations. Even so, dental disease is prevalent. The New England Elders Dental Study found the beginnings of periodontal disease in over 3/4 of the 1150 persons examined. Part of the problem, said these investigators, was that education and dental care for this population are overlooked by both dentists and the patients themselves (2).

The sad part of this situation is that proper dental hygiene and regular cleanings by the dentist are usually enough to stave off infection. Another simple and inexpensive way of preventing or at least halting the progression of periodontal disease is to store and replace your toothbrush properly. Although most of us are in the habit of keeping our toothbrush in the bathroom, this is not recommended. Bathrooms are the most contaminated room in the house. Healthy people should replace their toothbrushes every two weeks; those with a systemic or oral illness more often. Everyone should use a new toothbrush when they get sick, when they feel better and again when they completely recover (3).

Finally, an important aspect of both dental and general health is immunity. It has been determined that a suppressed immune system is associated with the rapid progression of periodontal disease. A

Midwestern research group found that cigarette smoking was one habit that dragged down immunity and sabotaged periodontitis treatment (4). Other lifestyle behaviors that theoretically could do the same include poor eating habits, stress and other immune depressors.

Myth No 3: The older I get, the sicker I'll get.

It's true that as we age, our physiology changes. These changes can lead to poor health if not addressed. But old age doesn't have to mean feeling sick and tired. An important part of staying well into the older years is keeping your immune system operating at its peak.

Aging is generally associated with lagging immunity and consequently more infections especially of the respiratory system. However John Hopkins' Professor Chandra discovered that when independent, apparently healthy, elderly people were fed nutritional supplements for a year, their immunity improved. Immunological responses were so marked that those who were supplemented (versus the placebo group) were plagued with less infections and took antibiotics for less days. It should be noted that these effects were achieved with a moderate amount of nutrients in a balanced formula; megadoses of some vitamins can actually impair immunity (5).

Besides taking care of your immunity with supplementation, diet, exercise and other measures, you can prevent many age-related diseases with specific health precautions. For example, there is evidence that smoking and low plasma levels of vitamins C and E, and beta-carotene contribute to cataracts (6). Dr. Dean Ornish showed that a one year program of stress management, moderate exercise, no smoking and a low-fat vegetarian diet may reverse the development of coronary atherosclerosis. Left untreated, atherosclerotic plagues usually continue to grow (7).

Many other chronic diseases can also be prevented or treated with lifestyle changes. Calcium and magnesium supplementation helps some individuals with hypertension. Most are helped by high potassium foods (fruits and vegetables), salt restriction and weight maintenance. Keeping blood pressure under control can also decrease the risk of a stroke.

Adult-onset diabetes is usually treated best with dietary measures such as reducing simple sugars, consuming a lot of fiber and taking chromium supplements (8). It's estimated that half of all types of cancer are linked to diet. This explains why less fat, lots of fruits, vegetables and fiber, vitamins A, B6, C and E and zinc and selenium all appear to play a role in cancer prevention (9).

Myth No 4: Lifestyle changes won't help me when I get old.

It's a mistaken notion that at a certain age, you reach the lifestyle modification point of no return. If you've used this as an excuse to cling to old, comfortable, unhealthy habits, it's time to let go. Of course, it's always best to live as healthy as possible as young as possible. But for those in their golden years, there's still plenty of hope.

Two of the most difficult habits to break, smoking and a sedentary lifestyle, can, when discarded, yield great health results. In 1990, the Surgeon General at that time, Antonia Novello, MD, MPH, declared that "even people who quit smoking at older ages can expect to enjoy a longer and healthier life compared with those who continue to smoke" (10).

Although the incidence of cigarette smoking naturally declines with age, those who continue to smoke should be aware of the numerous advantages of quitting. In as little as 20 minutes, blood pressure, pulse and body temperature all return to normal. Eight hours later, oxygen levels in the blood rise. After a day, the chance of a heart attack decreases. In five years, the risk of lung cancer falls to about half and in five more years lung cancer risk almost parallels that of a never-smoker (11). All these changes occur no matter what your age when you quit.

Frailty in the older person can't be totally blamed on aging. At least some weakness occurs because of physical inactivity. A regular exercise program not only decreases the risk of chronic illness, but can help prevent early death. Those who begin exercising later in life can slow or even reverse organ deterioration.

When elderly individuals exercise, they reap a number of health rewards. Aside from fighting chronic diseases, their heart is stronger, muscles are more fit and flexible, mood is enhanced, and falls and fractures are less frequent. While exercise alone probably doesn't significantly extend life beyond 80 years old, it can improve your quality of life (12,13).

Myth No 5: As long as I maintain the eating habits I had when I was younger, I'll stay healthy.

Perhaps one of the biggest fallacies of good health is that nutritional needs don't change with age. Just as children and teens have different dietary requirements than adults, so do the elderly differ in their needs from younger individuals.

A number of factors cause poor dietary intake. Chronic diseases, both physical and mental, can cause nutritional problems. Various medications can impair nutrient availability or discourage eating due to loss of appetite. If you wear ill-fitting dentures, pain can prevent you from eating. Elderly who live alone may feel isolated and uninterested in eating.

But even if you are older and healthy, the very process of aging alters your metabolism and physiology. Stomach acid declines, thus affecting some nutrient absorption. Many older people feel full sooner because of an increased sensitivity to the satiety peptide, cholecystokinin octapeptide. Aging also dampens the body's appetite center, and consequently eating. Finally, it's suspected that an older palate doesn't detect those tastes that drive us to the dinner table: salt and sweet (14).

Aging is inevitable. Poor health is not. Regular exercise, nutritious eating (appropriate for your age) and a lucky roll of the genetic dice can help you age with grace and good health.

References

1. Rosenberg IH, Miller JW. Nutritional factors in physical and cognitive functions of elderly people. American Journal of Clinical Nutrition 1992;55:1237S-43S.

2. Douglass CW et al. Oral health status of the elderly. New England Journal of Gerontology 1993;48(2):M39-M46.
3. Glass RT. The infected toothbrush, the infected denture, and transmission of disease: a review. Compendium of Continuing Education in Dentistry. 1992;13(8):592-9.
4. MacFarlane GD, Herzberg MC, Wolff LF, Hardie NA. Refractory periodontitis associated with abnormal polymorphonuclear leukocyte phagocytosis and cigarette smoking. Journal of Periodontology 1992;63(11):908-13.
5. Chandra RK. Effect of vitamin and trace-element supplementation on immune responses and infection in elderly subjects. The Lancet 1992;340:1124-27.
6. Harding JJ. Cigarette smoking and risk of cataracts (letter). Journal of the American Medical Association 1993;269(6):747.
7. Ornish D et al. Can lifestyle changes reverse coronary heart disease? The Lancet 1990;336:129-133.
8. Johnson K, Kligman E. Preventive nutrition: disease-specific dietary interventions for older adults. Geriatrics 1992;47(11):39-49.
9. Leis HP. The relationship of diet to cancer, cardiovascular disease and longevity. Internal Surgery 1991;76:1-5.
10. Novello AC. Surgeon General's report on the health benefits of smoking cessation. Public Health Reports 1990;105(6):545-48.
11. Timmreck TC, Randolph F. Smoking cessation: clinical steps to improve compliance. Geriatrics 1993;48(4):63-70.
12. Shephard RJ. Exercise and aging: extending independence in older adults. Geriatrics 1993;48(5):61-64.
13. Rooney EM. Exercise for older patients: why it's worth your effort. Geriatrics 1993;48(11):68-77.
14. Silver AJ. The malnourished older patient: when and how to intervene. Geriatrics 1993;48(7):70-74.

CHAPTER 13

R U STILL listening to your body?

There are 'early warning signs' that could be resolved with simple changes to diet or lifestyle. Many of these nutritional deficiencies or imbalances, if left, could result in serious illness or disease. Hamish MacGregor, a forensic scientist whose wife's craving for lettuce was the first sign she had breast cancer, wrote a book about physical symptoms and their causes. In his book, *The Body Language of Health*, he guides you to the exact supplement for your condition through targeted nutrition. The following are some of the signs, symptoms and associated deficient vitamins & minerals that he has discovered and documented.

Do you have dark rings under your eyes?

You may have an ALLERGY

What is an allergy?

An allergy is everything from a runny nose, itchy eyes and palate to skin rash. It aggravates the sense of smell, sight, tastes and touch causing irritation, extreme disability and sometimes fatality. It occurs when the body's immune system overreacts to normally harmless substances.

Allergy is widespread and affects approximately one in four of the population in the UK at some time in their lives. Each year the numbers are increasing by 5% with as many as half of all those affected being children.

What causes an allergy?

Allergic reactions are caused by substances in the environment known as allergens. Almost anything can be an allergen for someone. Allergens contain protein, which is often regarded as a constituent of the food we eat.

The most common allergens are pollen from trees and grasses, house dust mites, molds, pets such as cats and dogs, insects like wasps and bees, industrial and household chemicals, medicines, and foods such as milk and eggs.

Less common allergens include nuts, fruit and latex.

There are some non-protein allergens which include drugs such as penicillin. For these to cause an allergic response they need to be bound to a protein once they are in the body.

An allergic person's immune system believes allergens to be damaging and so produces a special type of antibody (IgE) to attack the invading material. This leads other blood cells to release further chemicals (including histamine) which together cause the symptoms of an allergic reaction.

The most common symptoms are: sneezing , runny nose, itchy eyes and ears, severe wheezing, coughing shortness of breath, sinus problems, a sore palate and nettle-like rash.

It should be understood that all the symptoms mentioned can be caused by factors other than allergy. Indeed some of the conditions are diseases in themselves.

Asthma, eczema, headaches, lethargy, loss of concentration and sensitivity to everyday foods represent a huge problem in society today.

Do you have Asthma?

You might have an allergy to MILK (also dust mite, pets, mold, pollen, other food allergies)

Asthma varies from inconvenient to irritating, debilitating or even life threatening.

Do you have Insomnia?

You may have a Vitamin B or a Mineral Deficiency.

Deficiencies in certain vitamins, minerals, amino acids and enzymes may disrupt sleep. Calcium, magnesium, B vitamins, folic acid and melatonin deficiencies may impair sleep.

What is insomnia?

Sometime in your life you may have difficulty sleeping—many people do. Anyone can suffer from insomnia, although sleeping problems are more common among women (especially menopausal), the ill, the elderly, smokers, and alcoholics. Sleep problems are, however, surprisingly common among young people. While it is not an illness and is in no way life-threatening, insomnia can be very distressing, frustrating, exhausting, depressing and at worst it can make you feel like you're going crazy.

Insomnia is either transitory (short term) or chronic (longer lasting). Problems sleeping take different forms:

- Difficulty falling asleep—more common among young people
- Sleeping lightly and restlessly, waking often, lying awake in the middle of the night—more common in people over 40. In younger people it may be associated with depression.
- Waking early and being unable to get back to sleep—this is more common in older people and anyone worrying about something in particular.

Do you have chronic fatigue syndrome?

If you do, you could be deficient in Molybdenum

Several studies report improvements in a number of underlying conditions with molybdenum (a trace mineral similar to Chromium). These conditions can often be misdiagnosed and hence can be given inappropriate medication. So supplementing with molybdenum is always worthwhile as it won't do any harm and may well do a lot of good.

For years, most physicians dismissed chronic fatigue syndrome (CFS) as an all-in-the-head problem. And most victims of CFS suffered the indignity of being told that they were hypochondriacs, and that they merely imagined their three main symptoms: (1) disabling fatigue; (2) persistent muscle and joint pain; and (3) severe problems of brain fog, irritability and depression.

Many doctors poured salt on the wounds of their patients by labeling their condition as, "yuppie syndrome", and a "syndrome created by the media". Fortunately that is all changing rapidly now.

What Is CFS? Chronic fatigue syndrome is a recent epidemic that can affect anybody of any age, suggesting it is a man-made ailment due to nutrition and lifestyle. CFS is a progressive immune disorder which affects all body organs and ecosystems. Thus, in addition to the three major symptoms of fatigue, muscle pain, and brain fog, most persons with severe CFS suffer from almost all of the following symptoms:

- Abdominal bloating, flatulence, and cramps (caused by battered bowel ecology)
- Digestive and absorptive problems (caused by damaged gastric ecology)
- Dizziness, lightheadedness, sweating, and weakness (due to oxidative stress on the blood ecology, itself caused by sugar-insulin-adrenaline roller coasters)
- Dry mouth, thirst and a sense of "toxicity" (caused by excessive detox stress on the liver ecology)

- Cold hands and feet, weight gain, and loss of hair (due to a sluggish thyroid)
- Chronic stress, irritability, and anxiety (due to relentless stress on the adrenal gland)
- Hypoglycemic symptoms (due to the instability of the pancreas)
- PMS, menstrual irregularities, lack of sex drive, and premature menopause (due to imbalance of sex hormones)
- Heart palpitations, low blood pressure, dizziness or sudden change of posture (due to oxidative stress on the cardiovascular system)
- Severe problems of mood, memory, and mentation problems (due to disruptions of neurotransmitters)
- Air or oxygen hunger due to sluggish oxygen transport and utilization)

People who tried molybdenum (a trace mineral similar to Chromium) for their condition reported the following:

Problem	Percentage who found improvement
Chronic Fatigue	*65%*
Chronic Weakness	*68%*
Joint Pain	*61%*
Muscle Pain	*61%*
Headaches	*55%*
Mental Concentration	*65%*
Memory	*71%*
Depression	*55%*
Insomnia	*61%*

Is your child disruptive and aggressive?

They may have a deficiency of zinc or vitamin B.

Children and adolescents with behavioral disorders and aggressive behavior are frequently malnourished. Those with certain nutritional deficiencies, such as those for zinc, iron, B vitamins and protein exhibit a 41% increase in aggressive behavior by the age of eight, and by the age of 17 there is violent and antisocial behavior in 51% (Am J Psychiatry 2004; 161: 2005-2013).

The deficiencies in the diet of these children resulted in abnormal development of the nervous system. Zinc is the single most common deficiency in the American population, with an estimated 80% of the whole population at risk. Zinc is important for many biological reactions and is especially significant in the maintenance of a healthy immune system. Zinc is also important in fetal development and specifically neurological function.

There is also evidence that iron deficiency may be an important contributor to the aggressive behavioral syndrome. Among adolescent males, iron deficiency has been shown to be directly associated with aggressive behavior (J Special Educ 1974; 8: 153-6). Moreover, in a population of imprisoned adolescents, the prevalence of iron deficiency was nearly twice that found in their non-incarcerated peers.

Vitamin B6 is essential for the synthesis or metabolism of practically all the neurotransmitters (chemicals which help to transmit messages in the nervous system). A deficiency of vitamin B6 causes symptoms such as tiredness, nervousness, irritability, depression and insomnia. In susceptible individuals it's not surprising that this deficiency can cause behavioral changes resulting in aggression and possibly criminal behavior (Crime Times 1997; 3: 6-7).

Protein is made up of amino acids, some of which are important in behavior. Some amino acids are precursors for neurotransmitters within the body. Certain proteins derived from the digestion of milk and wheat has drug-like effects that have the potential to affect neurotransmitters. Certain proteins have been shown scientifically to affect mood and behavior.

Do you produce excess ear wax?

If you do you may be deficient in ESSENTIAL FATTY ACIDS

Essential Fatty Acids, or EFA's are—well, as the name suggests—essential.

Excess ear wax is a classic symptom of deficiency in fatty acids, unless you actually have a troublesome ear infection.

Deficiency of EFA's can also cause dandruff.

Most people are deficient in EFA's. Our modern diet is lacking in the type of fats that are good for us, because the diet has been replaced with cheap oils and trans-fats that are indigestible and have little or no EFA content.

EFAs are also damaged by processing in the manufacture of cooking oils, margarines, shortenings, partially hydrogenated vegetable oils, trans fatty acids, and are also damaged by sautéing, frying, and deep-frying in food preparation. We need to get our EFA's from food, not fat and oil.

Essential fatty acids (EFAs) include linoleic acid and arachidonic acid, which are omega-6 (n-6) fatty acids, and linolenic acid, eicosapentaenoic acid, and docosahexaenoic acid, which are omega-3 (n-3) fatty acids. In the body, arachidonic acid can be made from linoleic acid, and eicosapentaenoic and docosahexaenoic acids can be made from linolenic acid.

EFAs are needed for many physiologic processes, including maintaining the integrity of the skin and the structure of cell membranes and synthesizing prostaglandins and leukotrienes. Eicosapentaenoic acid and docosahexaenoic acid are important components of the brain and retina.

Do your children have BEHAVIORAL AND LEARNING PROBLEMS?

Children with low blood levels of essential omega-3 fatty acids, have a greater tendency to have problems with behavior, learning and health consistent with attention deficit hyperactivity disorder (ADHD). Or maybe they're so stuffed up with ear wax they just can't hear you!!

Some previous studies by other researchers have indicated that symptoms associated with a deficiency in fatty acids are exhibited to a greater extent in children with ADHD. Those symptoms include thirst, frequent urination and dry skin and hair. Some researchers, however, were able to pinpoint omega-3s as the fatty acids that may be associated with the unique behavior problems in children with ADHD.

"There are two types of fatty acids that must be obtained from the foods we eat because the body cannot synthesize them," says John R. Burgess, assistant professor of foods and nutrition, Purdue University. "Omega-3 and omega-6 fatty acids are both essential to the body. However, evidence is accumulating that a deficiency of omega-3 fatty acids may be tied to behavior problems, learning and health problems."

ADHD is the most common behavioral disorder in children, affecting between 3 percent and 5 percent of school-age youngsters. It's diagnosed more often in boys than girls. The cause of ADHD is unknown, but research suggests many factors may contribute to it, including biological and environmental elements.

Stimulant drugs such as Ritalin often are used to calm children with ADHD and are effective about 75 percent of the time. "With our research we are trying to find potential causes of ADHD so that nutritional treatments can be developed for some children with ADHD," Burgess says.

Full-term babies fed a skim-milk formula low in linoleic acid may have growth failure, thrombocytopenia, alopecia, and a generalized scaly dermatitis, which resembles congenital ichthyosis, with increased water loss from the skin. This syndrome is reversed by linoleic acid supplementation. Deficiency is unlikely to occur on balanced diets, although cow's milk has only about 25% of the amount of linoleic acid in human milk. Although total fat intake in many developing countries is very low, much of the fat is of vegetable origin and is rich in linoleic acid with some linolenic acid.

Do you crave butter?

You probably have a deficiency in SODIUM

What is Sodium?

Sodium is a vital metallic element found at some level in nearly everything we eat. The body needs sodium to regulate blood pressure, blood volume, water balance and cell function. Salt regulates water retention in the body through the kidneys and adrenal glands. It is high in iodine, which is a mineral needed for thyroid function If you are craving salt, it may be your body asking for more iodine or potassium, or pointing to a fluid imbalance.

Are there any other symptoms of sodium deficiency?

It is possible to have a sodium deficiency resulting in symptoms such as severe muscle cramps, extreme weakness, and nausea. This is most likely to occur in people who are exercising long and hard in hot, humid weather. It can also happen as a result of severe vomiting or diarrhea. Laboratory studies with animals have revealed that severe deficiencies in sodium can result in very specific symptoms, and finally in death, due to the failure of renal function.

Excellent natural sources for sodium are celery, cucumbers & spirulina

Do you crave chocolate?

Cravings for *chocolate* may often be just your body crying out for *magnesium*.

Do you crave sugar, have blood sugar swings, or low blood sugar?

If you do, you may be deficient in CHROMIUM

Mostly, sugar craving is a metabolic dysfunction that may be due to imbalance of sugar and insulin. Chromium has a major effect on controlling the sugar balance in the body, and is deficient in our diet because refining foods removes the chromium. So if you crave sugar you're probably deficient in chromium, and scientists advise that you're probably heading for diabetes or insulin intolerance.

Sugar addiction

People who are addicted to sugar may be trying to treat their depression. Sugar addiction helps to beat depression, because it raises blood sugar levels, which in turn triggers the release of insulin. Insulin then pushes all nutrients, (including glucose into cells) leaving behind the larger molecules of tryptophan that is derived from food.

This is then converted to serotonin—our happiness hormone—in the presence of vitamin B6 and voila we feel happy. Thus the ingestion of sugar helps us to beat depression temporarily.

The trouble is that with continued consumption of excess sugar, receptors for insulin break down and become 'resistant to insulin'. If the insulin resistance is not treated, we will finish up with diabetes type II. High sugar consumption is also responsible for obesity, because high insulin (and stress hormones) interferes with the utilization of fat cells, and so we become fatter and fatter on sugar.

Do you crunch ice cubes or crave lettuce?

You could be iron deficient. Many iron-deficient patients develop pica, an unusual craving for specific foods (ice cubes, lettuce, etc.) that are often not even rich in iron.

Iron deficiency is the most common nutritional disorder in the world. The numbers are staggering: as many as **4-5 billion people,** 66-80% of the world's population, may be iron deficient; 2 billion people—over 30% of the world's population—are anemic, mainly due to iron deficiency, and in developing countries, the condition is frequently exacerbated by malaria and worm infections.

Iron deficiency affects more people than any other condition, constituting a public health condition of epidemic proportions. More subtle in its manifestations than, for example, protein-energy malnutrition, it exacts the heaviest overall toll in terms of ill-health, premature death and lost earnings.

Iron deficiency and anemia reduce the work capacity of individuals and entire populations, bringing serious economic consequences and obstacles to national development. Conversely, treatment can raise national productivity levels by 20%.

Overall, it is the most vulnerable, the poorest and the least educated who are disproportionately affected by iron deficiency, and it is they who stand to gain the most by its reduction.

The symptoms of iron deficiency are those normally associated with anemia itself (easy fatigue, rapid heart rate, palpitations and rapid breathing on exertion.

Severe iron deficiency causes progressive skin and mucosal changes. These include a smooth tongue and brittle nails.

Do you or your family have a history of cancer?

If you do, you may be deficient in SELENIUM

Our bodies need selenium, an antioxidant that might help control cell damage that can lead to cancer.

The Nutritional Prevention of Cancer Trial included 1,300 men and women. Men who had taken selenium for 6½ years had approximately 60 percent fewer new cases of prostate cancer than men who took the placebo. In 2002, study data showed that men who took selenium for more than 7½ years had about 52 percent fewer new cases of prostate cancer than men who took the placebo.

A deficiency in the mineral selenium is associated with many types of cancer, while the presence of a chemical found in some vegetables (sulforaphane) is known have a powerful role in cancer prevention.

Recent research on human cancer genes has found that foods that contain the mineral selenium and plant-based chemical sulforaphane in combination may have a 13 times greater ability to protect against cancer than when the food compounds are used separately.

Selenium is a mineral that is found in nuts, poultry, fish, eggs, sunflower seeds and mushrooms. Having a deficiency of selenium in the diet is known to be associated with a number of cancers, including prostate cancer.

Sulforaphane is being investigated as a potential cancer drug. It is found in foods such as broccoli, sprouts, cabbage, watercress and lettuce.

People who have deficiencies often develop a craving. Did her body know? Was it craving for sulforaphane or iron which is also *found in lettuce*? We'll never know. But with all my research I have not come across any other reference to lettuce in this way.

Take notice of your cravings. They mean something. Pregnant women can crave the strangest things—coal, soil, oranges, pizza. Your body has decided it needs whatever these products contain.

Vitamin E for prostate cancer prevention?

We get vitamin E in a wide range of foods, especially vegetables, vegetable oils, nuts, and egg yolks. Vitamin E, like selenium, is an antioxidant, which might help control cell damage that can lead to cancer.

In a 1998 study of 29,100 male smokers in Finland, men who took vitamin E to prevent lung cancer had 32 percent fewer new cases of prostate cancer than men who took the placebo.

Do you bite your nails?

You may be deficient in MINERALS

What are minerals?

Yes, nail biting often begins with boredom or impatience or fidgeting.

If you are among the millions who regularly bite their nails, you've probably said to yourself "I *wish* I could stop biting my nails!"

But often your body needs the minerals in the nail material that your body is recycling. So the reward-cycle begins and continues.

Studies show that the mineral content of hair or nails is similar to the mineral content of bone.

The human body, like everything else in nature, is made up of chemicals.

Since the trace minerals group includes over 50 chemical elements, scientists further subdivide this group into three categories, in order to separate the minerals that are important in health from others that are in our bodies just because they are in the environment and probably have no special role.

The first category is the essential trace minerals. These are minerals that are required in the diet for full health, and when the intake is insufficient, symptoms of deficiency will arise. They include nine known to be essential: zinc, copper, selenium, chromium, manganese, molybdenum, iodine, fluoride, and cobalt. About 10 more minerals are thought to be essential but the full proof is not yet in; these are arsenic, boron, bromine, cadmium, lead, lithium, nickel, silicon, tin, and vanadium. You will note in this list several minerals (arsenic, cadmium, lead) that are normally thought to be toxic.

This leads to the second category of trace minerals, the toxic trace minerals. The term is used for minerals that give problems with toxicity at levels that may be encountered normally in the environment and for which health concerns are more likely to arise from too much rather than too little in the body. This category is fairly loose, changing from time to time, and includes aluminum, arsenic, cadmium, lead, mercury, and tin.

Actually, all nutrients are toxic if too much is ingested; how much is too much depends on the nutrient. For essential minerals like copper, there is a definite gradation for health; if the intake is below the requirement, illness due to deficiency will develop; as the intake goes up, health will improve until a plateau is reached, where small increases in intake will not make any difference to health; above the top safe level (the end of the plateau), increases in intake will cause toxic illness. In extreme cases, both deficiency at one end and toxicity at the other end of the spectrum may get so severe as to cause death. This pattern is seen for all nutrients, including, for example, vitamins, macro-minerals, and protein.

Some will cause debilitating disease. A classic example is vanadium which can cause manic depression.

The third category of nonessential trace minerals is everything else: all the other minerals that are present in the body but are not essential in the diet and are not thought to have any function, and that do not cause any concern over toxicity or deficiency. In practice, virtually everything is essential.

Biting your nails becomes addictive because of the reward process. You're probably deficient in minerals.

Do you suffer from soft or brittle nails?

You may be deficient in MAGNESIUM

What is Magnesium?
Magnesium functions in more than 300 enzymatic reactions. Magnesium is essential for the conversion of vitamin D to its biologically active form that then helps the body absorb and utilize the calcium. The typical Western diet is frequently very low in magnesium. Many surveys have indicated that over 80 percent of Americans get less than

the Recommended Dietary Intake (RDI) of this important mineral. The highest magnesium concentration is found in the tissues that are most metabolically active including the brain, heart, liver, and kidney.

"Every 30 seconds someone will die from cardiovascular disease." Magnesium supplements can improve energy production within the heart, improve delivery of oxygen to the heart, reduce demand on the heart, inhibit the formation of blood clots, and improve heart rate. "Magnesium supplementation has been used in many of these applications for over 50 years!"

Magnesium is also effective with Chronic Fatigue Syndrome. People with CFS have low red blood cell magnesium levels. A recent study in the United Kingdom conducted a double-blind experiment with CFS patients and magnesium supplements. The researchers concluded that 80% of the patients receiving magnesium reported "significantly improved energy levels, better emotional state, and less pain."

On a daily average, more than 9 million Western people are exposed to noise levels above 85 decibels, the level where the risk for permanent hearing loss increases exponentially. Since magnesium is essential in regulating cellular membrane permeability and neuromuscular excitability, researchers decided to test the hypothesis that noise-induced hearing loss and magnesium are related. The researchers were right! They discovered that magnesium supplementation is highly effective in preventing noise-induced hearing loss.

General Brittle Nails Information

Brittle nails are characterized by splitting or breaking at the nail tip. The nail can also appear as thin, shiny, dry or translucent. The nails can reveal much about a person's general internal health, so nail abnormalities in either the fingers or toes can indicate an underlying disorder.

Possible Causes of Brittle Nails

Brittle nails are often caused by nutritional deficiencies or underlying medical conditions.

Possible Lifestyle Changes for Brittle Nails

Eat a diet high in whole grains, fresh fruits and vegetables, legumes, oatmeal, nuts and seeds. Drink plenty of water and fresh fruit juices. Take two tablespoons of brewer's yeast or wheat germ oil daily. Avoid refined sugars and simple carbohydrates. Apply a mixture of equal parts honey, avocado oil, egg yolk and a pinch of salt to your nails to restore color and texture. Treat nails gently and protect them from hot water and harmful chemicals by wearing protective gloves. Do not pick or pull on the nails. Wear a protective base coat to help strengthen nails.

Magnesium plays important roles in the structure and the function of the human body. The adult human body contains about 25 grams of magnesium. Over 60% of all the magnesium in the body is found in the skeleton, about 27% is found in muscle, while 6 to 7% is found in other cells, and less than 1% is found outside of cells

Magnesium is involved in more than 300 essential metabolic reactions. The metabolism of carbohydrates and fats to produce energy requires numerous magnesium-dependent chemical reactions. Magnesium is required by the adenosine triphosphate synthesizing protein in mitochondria. ATP, the molecule that provides energy for almost all metabolic processes, exists primarily as a complex with magnesium (MgATP). Magnesium is required at a number of steps during the synthesis of nucleic acids (DNA and RNA) and proteins. A number of enzymes participating in the synthesis of carbohydrates and lipids require magnesium for their activity. Glutathione, an important antioxidant, requires magnesium for its synthesis. Magnesium plays a structural role in bone, cell membranes, and chromosomes.

Early **signs of magnesium deficiency** include loss of appetite, nausea, vomiting, fatigue, and weakness. As magnesium deficiency worsens, numbness, tingling, muscle contractions and cramps, seizures, personality changes, abnormal heart rhythms, and coronary spasms can occur. Severe magnesium deficiency can result in low levels of calcium in the blood (hypocalcemia). Magnesium deficiency is also associated with low levels of potassium in the blood (hypokalemia)

Are you craving chocolate? Then your body wants magnesium!

Magnesium Sources

Water
Many water supplies, both public and private, contain small doses of magnesium. For a larger dose of the mineral, try drinking hard or mineral water. Soft water will contain the smallest dose.

Vegetables
Many vegetables contain magnesium, but leafy greens are your best source. Try some spinach, swiss chard or beet greens for a high dose of the mineral. Artichokes, okra, parsnips, sweet potatoes, potatoes and squash are also great sources.

Meat
When it comes to eating meat with high magnesium, you want to look to fish. Halibut and tuna are the front runners, providing a mega dose of magnesium.

Fruit
A few types of fruit offer a decent amount of magnesium, such as bananas and dried figs.

Beans
Beans are a fantastic source of magnesium, and a wide array of the food contains high doses of the mineral. Try anything from black, navy or white beans to lima, pinto and soy beans. Peas and kidney beans also provide a fair amount of magnesium.

Whole Grains
Whole grains are yet another great source of magnesium. Buckwheat, oat bran, cornmeal, barley and wheat are all helpful for getting your daily dose of the mineral.

Nuts and Seeds

Most nuts and seeds contain at least a small amount of magnesium, but almonds, pumpkin seeds, cashews and pine nuts offer the highest doses.

Do you suffer from hypertension?

If you do, you may be deficient in MAGNESIUM (see soft or brittle nails)

Do you suffer from high blood pressure?

If you do, you may be deficient in MAGNESIUM

An observational study examined the effect of various nutritional factors on incidence of high blood pressure in over 30,000 US male health professionals. After four years of follow-up, it was found that a lower risk of hypertension was associated with dietary patterns that provided more magnesium, potassium, and dietary fiber.

Many healthcare professionals are realizing that blood pressure tablets are wrongly targeted for many people, and can cause undesirable side effects.

Magnesium and diabetes

In recent years, rates of type 2 diabetes have increased along with the rising rates of obesity.

Magnesium plays an important role in carbohydrate metabolism. It may influence the release and activity of insulin, the hormone that helps control blood glucose (sugar) levels. Low blood levels of magnesium are frequently seen in individuals with type 2 diabetes.

Low magnesium may worsen insulin resistance, a condition that often precedes diabetes. The kidneys will excrete magnesium during periods of severe hyperglycemia (significantly elevated blood glucose).

In older adults, correcting magnesium depletion may improve insulin response and action.

One health study followed over 170,000 health professionals through diet questionnaires. Over time, the risk for developing type 2 diabetes was greater in men and women with a lower magnesium intake.

Do you have stretch marks?

You may be deficient in ZINC

What is Zinc?

Many of the features of common chronic disorders, especially connective tissue disorders, are identical to the symptoms of zinc deficiencies. Is this a coincidence, or could zinc deficiencies be an often overlooked factor in many disorders currently attributed to genes or other causes?

Do you have chicken skin on your upper arms?

If you do, you may be deficient in ESSENTIAL FATTY ACIDS

Keratosis pilaris (KP) is a very common genetic follicular disease that is manifested by the appearance of rough bumps on the skin and hence colloquially referred to as "chicken skin". Primarily, it appears on the back and outer sides of the upper arms, but can also occur on thighs and buttocks or any body part except palms or soles.

Full-term babies fed a skim-milk formula low in linoleic acid may have growth failure, thrombocytopenia, alopecia, and a generalized scaly dermatitis, which resembles congenital ichthyosis, with increased water loss from the skin. This syndrome is reversed by linoleic acid supplementation. Deficiency is unlikely to occur on balanced diets, although cow's milk has only about 25% of the amount of linoleic acid in human milk. Although total fat intake in many developing countries is very low, much of the fat is of vegetable origin and is rich in linoleic acid with some linolenic acid.

Do you often have cold hands and feet?

You might have a deficiency in **MAGNESIUM (see above)**

Do you have shaking hands?

If you do, you could be deficient in MAGNESIUM and VITAMIN B1

Early symptoms of magnesium deficiency can include fatigue, anorexia, irritability, insomnia, and **muscle tremors** or twitching.

People only slightly deficient in magnesium become irritable, high-strung, sensitive to noise, hyperexcitable, apprehensive, and belligerent. If the deficiency is more severe, or prolonged, they may develop twitching, tremors, irregular pulse, insomnia, muscle weakness, jerkiness, and leg and foot cramps; their hands may shake so badly that their writing becomes illegible.

Electroencephalograms, electrocardiograms, and electromyograms, or the records of electrical waves in the brain, heart, and muscles, all become abnormal.

If magnesium is severely deficient, the brain is particularly affected. Clouded thinking, confusion, disorientation, marked depression, and even terrifying hallucinations of delerium tremens are largely brought on by a lack of this nutrient and remedied when magnesium is given.

Improvement is usually dramatic within hours after magnesium is taken.

If shaking or trembling has been present for less than two years, it may be caused by temporary conditions such as:

- Increased anxiety or stress

- Certain medications
- Caffeine excess or caffeine withdrawal
- Nicotine or smoking excess or nicotine withdrawal

Alcohol excess or alcohol/drug withdrawal such as shaking or trembling could also be caused by conditions such as:

- Endocrine imbalances
- Electrolyte imbalances
- Hormonal imbalances

As many as one in 20 people older than age 40 and one in five people over 65 may have essential tremor (ET). There may be as many as 10 million people with ET in the United States, and many more worldwide. Essential tremor is much more common than most neurologic disease, with the exception of stroke, and is more common than Parkinson's disease—a disorder characterized by resting tremor, stiffness and slowness of movement.

Essential tremor is a very common but complex neurologic movement disorder. It's called "essential" because in the past, it had no known cause. It's not caused by another neurological condition or the side effect of a medication. ET usually affects the hands, but it may also affect the head and neck (causing shaking), face, jaw, tongue, voice (causing a shaking or quivering sound), the trunk and, rarely, the legs and feet. The tremor may be a rhythmic "back-and-forth" or "to-and-fro" movement produced by involuntary (unintentional) contractions of the muscle. Severity of the tremors can vary greatly from hour to hour and day to day.

Some people experience tremor only in certain positions—this is called postural tremor. Tremor that worsens while writing or eating is called kinetic or action-specific tremor. Most people with ET have both postural and kinetic tremor.

Vitamin B1 is a water-soluble vitamin needed to process carbohydrates, fat, and protein. Every cell of the body requires vitamin

B1 to form the fuel the body runs on—adenosine triphosphate (ATP). Nerve cells require vitamin B1 in order to function normally. Deficiency can cause tremors.

A decline in vitamin B1 levels occurs with age, irrespective of medical condition. Deficiency is most commonly found in alcoholics, people with poor absorption conditions, and those eating a very poor diet. It is also common in children with congenital heart disease. People with chronic fatigue syndrome may also be deficient in vitamin B1. Individuals undergoing regular kidney dialysis may develop severe vitamin B1 deficiency, which can result in serious complications.

Do you have a white coating on your tongue?

You might be dehydrated or you could have a yeast infection.

Water requirements:

Current recommendations for water are eight, eight-ounce glasses per day which would equal 64 ounces. This amount should be sufficient for most healthy persons who are not in a hot, humid environment or sweating from physical work or exercise and should drink more water more often. Drink water, not soft drinks which are loaded with sugar.

Hot countries in the world happen to have the worst water supplies. Many women walk over ten miles a day (15 kilometers) just to get water.

It is easier to pay attention to the color of your urine each time you urinate. (Urine that has accumulated in your bladder during sleep will be more concentrated and yellow. Otherwise, if your kidneys didn't concentrate urine during sleep, you would have to wake up to urinate.) After urinating the first time after waking up, your urine should be light colored and odorless for the remainder of the day. This assumes that you have normal functioning kidneys and no bladder disease or infection.

Some foods will affect urine smell and color. For example, asparagus produces a strange smell to your urine, due to methylthioacrylate and methylthiopropionate from the asparagus. Turmeric turns the urine bright yellow.

Do you rub your eyes ?

You could have a stress or sleep problem

When you rub your eyes it stimulates the ocularcardio reflex, applying pressure around the rectus muscles that move the eyeball. This causes a response in the vagus nerve, through their close association.

This stimulation lowers heart rate, so we rub our eyes in order to slow ourselves down to prepare to sleep. Producing a vagal response in this manner (sometimes to the degree of inducing a faint) is used in martial arts, massage, hypnotism, and is a method of disabling violent prisoners/patients.

For some people, this feels good. and may be one reason why stressed people sometimes gain benefit from rubbing their eyes and face with their hands, especially after a stressful telephone call, meeting or confrontation.

Eyes and allergies

Many people with eye rubbing problems have dry eyes that can be associated with an allergy. The more inflamed the tissue gets, the more it itches—this is called the itch/scratch/itch cycle that doesn't stop until damage has been done.

Do you have hemorrhoids (or piles)?

You may have a deficiency of fiber in your diet.

What are hemorrhoids?

Hemorrhoids (also known as piles) are rather like varicose veins in the canal of the anus. Here, just under the mucous membrane (inner lining), is a considerable network of veins extending upwards for an inch or so from the level of the skin to just above the anal canal, where it joins the rectum. When the veins of this network become swollen with blood, hemorrhoids occur.

The vein swelling can affect the part of the network just above the anal canal, where it is less well supported by the muscular ring (sphincter), and this causes internal hemorrhoids. Or it may affect the veins at the lower end of the canal, just under the skin, causing external hemorrhoids. Some people have both.

Hemorrhoids are a common problem and affect around 50% of people at some time in their life. Although uncomfortable and embarrassing, it is not normally a serious condition.

The common symptoms of hemorrhoids are:

- Itching around the anus
- Signs of blood (bright red) on toilet paper after a bowel motion
- Soreness and discomfort during and immediately after a bowel motion
- A visible swelling around the anus
- A feeling that your bowels have not been completely emptied

Sometimes hemorrhoids inside the anal canal protrude outside the anus. These are known as prolapsed or prolapsing hemorrhoids. At first, the hemorrhoid may go back in by itself, but later you might need to push it back in yourself using your finger.

Protruding hemorrhoids can lead to skin irritation and discomfort and there is usually mucus discharge from the irritated mucous membrane. Hemorrhoids can become inflamed and swollen, but are rarely very painful, unless associated with an actual splitting of the anus (anal fissure).

Hemorrhoids are thought to be caused by constipation. If you have constipation over a period of time and often have to strain to pass hard stools, this can damage the lining of the anal canal. If this happens often enough, the veins may lose their normal support and protection. Some people are thought to have veins especially liable to this kind of injury. This is probably just a matter of chance anatomical variation.

Hemorrhoids are not caused by sitting on cold hard surfaces, prolonged standing or sedentary work.

Do you frequently catch colds and other respiratory infections?

If you do, you may be deficient in VITAMIN C and ZINC

Reviews of the research conducted on the use of Vitamin C over the past 20 years conclude that, in general, large doses of vitamin C have been found to **decrease the duration and severity** of colds, an effect that may be related to the antihistamine effects found to occur with large doses (eg two grams) of vitamin C. But large doses of vitamin C do not have a significant effect on the **number of colds** you catch, except for certain susceptible groups (e.g., individuals with low dietary intake, and athletes) who may be less susceptible to the common cold when taking supplemental vitamin C.

One aspect of human physiology which points towards a diet heavily reliant on fruit and vegetables, rather than meat, is our **lack of ability to synthesize vitamin C.**

Humans and only one or two mammalian species cannot manufacture vitamin C, one of the most important vitamins. This suggests that long ago we existed on a diet of fruit and vegetables, high in vitamin C, and therefore didn't need the ability to manufacture it. Now, vitamin C is one of the main supplements taken in Western societies.

Deficiency in vitamin C has more serious implications. Vitamin C is required for the synthesis of collagen, an important structural component of blood vessels, tendons, ligaments, and bone. Vitamin C also plays an important role in the synthesis of neurotransmitters that are critical to brain function and are known to affect mood.

Recent research also suggests that vitamin C is involved in the metabolism of cholesterol to bile acids which may have implications for blood cholesterol levels and the incidence of gallstones.

A large number of studies have shown that increased consumption of fresh fruits and vegetables is associated with a reduced risk for most types of cancer. Such studies are the basis for dietary guidelines endorsed by the U.S. Department of Agriculture and the National Cancer Institute, which recommend at least five servings of fruits and vegetables per day. A number of case-control studies have investigated the role of vitamin C in cancer prevention. Most have shown that higher intakes of vitamin C are associated with decreased incidence of cancers of the mouth, throat and vocal chords, esophagus, stomach, colorectal, and lung.

BUT if you get a cold, don't guzzle orange juice for the vitamin C it contains. A big dose of sugar is what you'd actually be getting, making you even more ill. You'll conclude that you must not have caught the illness in time, which couldn't have been any further from the truth. The sugar simply fed your infection. If you want that much vitamin C, take a vitamin pill, washed down with plenty of water. Your body is 70 percent water—and that is exactly what it needs!

Sufficient zinc is also essential in maintaining immune system function.

Statistics & Fun Facts

- The USDA's food intake surveys show that the food-away-from-home sector provided 32 percent of total food energy consumption in 1994-96. It has now risen to 47 percent and continues to rise.
- Exercisers feel sick almost 30% less often than non-exercisers
- In the U.S., survey data from the Department of Agriculture has shown that 52% of our overall vegetable consumption comes from iceberg lettuce, potatoes and canned tomatoes.
- Heart disease & cancer continue to be the leading killers of men and women alike.

- Over three decades ago, people averaged eight to nine hours of sleep each night. Today, many people only sleep six to seven hours. In order to keep up energy levels, people are turning to food. Studies have shown that those who are sleep deprived ingest as much as 10-15 percent more calories.
- Research from Oxford University shows exercising in groups releases feel-good endorphins in the brain.
- Tongue prints are as unique as finger prints.
- The human brain weights three pounds and is 90 percent water.
- There are 206 bones in the human body and 1/4 or 51 of them are in your feet.
- 70-80% of overweight children become overweight adults.
- Obese parents are 60-70% more likely to have obese children.
- You spend one third of your lifetime sleeping, which is twenty years in an average lifetime.
- Your heart is the strongest muscle of your body, beating about 100,000 times in one day in an average adult.
- Your tongue is actually a collection of muscles; proportional to their size. They're also the strongest muscles in your body.
- The human nervous system can relay messages to the brain at speeds of up to 200 miles per hour. Your brain receives 100 million nerve messages each second from your senses.
- From all the oxygen that a human breathes, only twenty percent goes to the brain.
- Saffron, which is made from dried stamens of crocus flowers, is the world's most expensive spice.
- There are hundreds to thousands of varieties of a single fruit or vegetable. For instance, there are 7,500 plants worldwide. The United States grows 2,500 of these, but just 100 of them are grown commercially.
- Women blink twice as often as men.
- Men sweat more than women.
- Human thighbones are stronger than concrete.

- Although the outside of a bone is hard, they are generally light and soft inside. Bones are also about 75% water.
- Approximately two-thirds of a person's body weight is water. Blood is 92% water. The brain is 75% water and muscles are 75% water.
- The body carries about 25 trillion red blood cells (erythrocytes), the most abundant cells in the body. Red blood cells make up about 45% of blood's volume.
- The average life of a taste bud is 10 days.
- Half your body's red blood cells are replaced every seven days. Coconut water can be used (in emergencies) as a substitute for blood plasma. The reason for this is that coconut water (the water found in coconuts—not to be confused with coconut milk, which comes from the flesh of the coconut) is sterile and has an ideal pH level. Coconut water is liquid endosperm—it surrounds the embryo and provides nutrition.
- Laughing lowers levels of stress hormones and strengthens the immune system. Six-year-olds laugh an average of 300 times a day. Adults only laugh 15 to 100 times a day.

Top 10 best-selling grocery items

Carbonated drinks ($12 billion in sales)
Milk ($11b)
Bread & rolls ($9b)
Beer/ale ($8b)
Salty snacks ($8b)
Cheese ($7b)
Frozen dinners ($6b)
Cold cereal ($6b)
Wine ($5b)
Cigarettes ($4b)

Conclusion

Now that I have given you my Four-Pillar system and specifically shown you how to reverse, retrain, rebuild your body & mind using the R3 Diet, the ball is in your court. R3FitWorld.com is available for you to have ongoing online guidance, support and accountability. It is now up to you to make a resolute statement such as, "I will get the things I need to prepare myself for success and start R3 immediately" or something as simple as, "I'm in". Our bodies are amazing and you will be amazed at how quickly it responds to the right foods. Do not allow any of your mind's justifications to talk you out of it. I would like to conclude by giving you my golden rules that have helped me and my clients stick to R3 until you can confidently say, "R3 for life!"

Golden Rule #1: NEVER compromise/substitute anything on the R3 Diet during Mon-Thurs & ALWAYS have at least two R3 meals each day Fri-Sun.

Golden Rule #2: One compromise leads to an ambush of compromises, which leads to the whole thing being compromised. So just say NO to that first thought that asks you to compromise no matter how small.

Golden Rule #3: When you first think of water you don't think drown, you think thirst quencher & you know it provides hydration. So when you first think of food, don't think burden or evil, think medicine & know that it provides a long, limitless, lovely, lively life!

CHAPTER 14

R U ready to eat?

Juice Recipes

Reveal Juice

6-8 pears, washed well, core and seeds intact

1/2-inch fresh gingerroot, peeled

1/4 cup fresh parsley, washed well

Relief Juice

1/2 Medium fresh beetroot

3 Broccoli Stalks

½ Red Pepper

2 Tomatoes

Dash Tabasco sauce

Reward Ginger Ale

2 Apples, cored and sliced

1 Lemon

1 Lime

1/2 inch fresh Ginger

Handful of Grapes

Sparkling mineral water

Required Juice

    1 cup of spinach
    1 cucumber
    2 stalks of celery including leaves
    3 carrots
    1 apple

Repair Juice

    ½ head of Cabbage
    2 Apples

Reset Juice

    3 Cucumbers
    2 Apples
    2 Garlic Cloves
    1 handful Parsley

Recoup Melonade

    ½ Watermelon (discard rind)
    2 Lemons (discard rind)
    ¼ cup of Mint Leaves

SMOOTHIE RECIPES

Refresh Smoothie

    Bok Choy
    Oranges
    Red Grapefruit
    Strawberries
    Sour Apples

Remember Smoothie
Spinach
Raspberries
Blueberries

Recharge Smoothie
Kale
Swiss Chard
Bananas
Grapes

Reclaim Smoothie
Celery
Bananas
Apples
Tsp Cinnamon

Reduce Smoothie
Collard Greens
Pears
Kiwi

Rejoice Smoothie
Lacinato Kale
Bananas
Papaya
Dates

Relax Smoothie
Rainbow Chard
Mango
Peaches

Fruit Meals

R U Happy?
Bananas

R U Youthful?
Blueberries
Raspberries
Strawberries

R U Radiant?
Kiwi
Sweet Plums

R U Hydrated?
Melon
Cantaloupe

R U Ripped?
Grapefruit
Pineapple
Oranges

R U Healthy?
Bananas
Grapes

R U Pain—Free?
Apples
Cherries

Salads

Rawsome
Spinach
Walnuts
Oranges

Rawk On
Romaine
Black Beans
Tomatoes
Onions
Cilantro

Rawsistable
Cucumbers
Tomatoes
Corn
Avocados
Italian Parsley

Rawnowned
Red Cabbage
Diced Beets
Cucumber
Scallions
Served w/Tomato Soup

Rawpresent
Endive
Yellow Pepper

Celery

Garlic

Tarragon w/Whole-Grain Toast

Rawvolution

Broccoli

Onions

Raisins

Sunflower Seeds

Rawsolve

Massaged Kale

Shredded Carrots

Radishes

Shallots

Avocado

Notes

~The following section is designated for the cooked recipes. I mention sautéing vegetables in many recipes. The amount will be based on your household. However you want to ensure satiety of each family member. When in doubt, think 1-3 handfuls of the sautéed vegetables on each individual plate.

~I mention Extra Virgin Olive Oil (EVOO) in most of the meals for simplicity; however you should rotate your favorite healthy oil ie. coconut oil, grapeseed oil, flax seed oil & hemp seed oil & avocado oil etc.

~I mention the 3 specific brands on the following pages:

1. Braggs Vinaigrette-It is a dressing that can be purchased at your local health food store.
2. Arrowhead Mills Buttermilk Pancake & Waffle Mix-It can also be purchased at your local health food store.
3. Ezekiel Wraps are available in the frozen sections of local health food stores and some chain grocery stores.

Protein Meals

Remarkable Baked Tuna Steaks

Bake fresh tuna steaks in oiled aluminum foil topped with lemon, pepper & capers in oven at 375° for 12 minutes.

Serve with sautéed broccoli, yellow squash & thyme.

Robust Sautéed Scallops

Sautee scallops EVOO, garlic, pepper, fennel seeds until well done.

Serve with sautéed spinach, tomatoes,& onions

Rosemary Shrimp Delight

Sauté shrimp in EVOO, garlic & rosemary.

Serve with steamed yellow squash, zucchini, celery& rosemary.

Rustic Teriyaki Fish

Dredge fish (salmon or halibut) lightly with wheat germ. In a large skillet, heat a generous amount of EVOO, and sauté fish until browned on both sides. Add sliced celery and scallions and sauté a few minutes longer. Mix wine vinegar and nama shoyu (or low sodium soy sauce) and dry mustard in a bowl and pour over fish in the skillet. Lower heat, and simmer gently for 10 minutes.

Serve with steamed snow peas, bean sprouts and carrots, and fresh tarragon

Rich Chipotle-Glazed Chicken

Preheat oven to 400°. In a small bowl, mix an even amount each of: chipotle chilies, garlic, honey, apple cider vinegar, cumin, and cinnamon to make a paste. Rub the paste evenly over each breast. Place the chicken breasts on an EVOO greased pan and bake until the chicken is just cooked through, about 25 to 30 minutes. Serve garnished with cilantro.

Serve with sautéed turnip greens, yellow peppers, red pepper flakes, shallots, oregano, onion powder & lemon juice.

Regal Shrimp & Asparagus Stir-Fry

Sautee shrimp, asparagus, water chestnuts & grated ginger in sesame oil for 6 minutes.

Stir in nama shoyu (or low sodium soy sauce), lime and serve.

Revamped Eggplant Parmesan

Ingredients:
Eggplants
fresh garlic
fresh basil
dried oregano
tomato pasta sauce (preferably homemade, but premade is OK)
mozzarella cheese
parmesan cheese
Brussels sprouts—side dish

Preheat oven to 350°. Oil baking pan with EVOO. Cut the unpeeled eggplants into ½ inch rounds. Arrange eggplant rounds in the pan, drizzle with olive oil and add fresh garlic & basil along with dried oregano. Bake approximately 20 minutes, until eggplant begins to soften. Pour (preferably homemade) tomato pasta sauce over eggplant, return to oven for 10 minutes. Cover with mozzarella and Parmesan and place under broiler until cheese is nicely melted and browning.

Serve with steamed Brussels sprouts that have been sautéed in butter, garlic & cracked pepper.

Carb Meals

Really Colorful Pasta
    Whole grain pasta of choice
    Fresh garlic
    Yellow pepper
    Diced tomatoes
    Broccoli
    Cauliflower
    Onions
    Dried cumin
    Tomato pasta sauce (preferably homemade)
    Parsley for garnish

Reach in your carb pantry and choose a whole-grain pasta in the shape you prefer: penne, bow ties, elbows, spaghetti, angel hair or linguini, etc. Bring water to a boil in your rice cooker & then add EVOO and pasta. Check the package for approx cook times. Meanwhile, place some EVOO in a wok and sauté your garlic, yellow peppers, diced tomatoes, broccoli, cauliflower, onions & sprinkle with cumin. Pour (preferably homemade) tomato pasta sauce over vegetables in wok. Drain your pasta and plate it with your vegetables & sauce and garnish with parsley.

Really Spicy Beans & Lentils

Three varieties of beans/lentils (must be pre-soaked overnight)
Fresh garlic
Shredded carrots
Celery
Red pepper
Diced tomatoes
Cayenne
Cumin
Oregano
Turmeric

Reach in your carb pantry and choose three of the beans/lentils you prefer: black beans, mung beans, red lentils, green lentils, etc. (Remember to soak beans overnight) Bring water to a boil in your rice cooker & then add EVOO. **Make sure to use twice as much water to beans.** Meanwhile, saute garlic, shredded carrots, celery, red pepper, diced tomatoes, cayenne, cumin, oregano & turmeric in your wok. Add the beans & lentils to your vegetables.

Serve with this healthy cornbread recipe: Preheat oven to 325°. Lightly grease a muffin pan. Combine ½ cup of cornmeal, ½ cup whole-wheat flour, ½ tsp baking soda, and ½ tsp sea salt in a large bowl; stir in ½ cup of applesauce, ½ cup of rice or hemp milk, and ¼ cup of agave nectar. Slowly add 2 TBSP of oil while stirring. Pour the mixture into the muffin pan. Bake for 15 to 20 minutes.

Really Smothered Baked Potato

Pre-heat oven to 400°. Place unwrapped potatoes on an ungreased pan & bake for 30 minutes or until done. Meanwhile, sauté garlic, spinach, corn, onions, chives & rosemary. Put a pat of butter on baked potato and smother with sautéed vegetables. Garnish with black olives and/or jalepenos.

Really Stuffed Zucchini

Preheat oven to 400°.

Ingredients:
Brown rice vermicelli OR whole grain angel hair pasta (Make enough to fill the zucchinis. Amount will vary according to size of zucchinis.)
2-3 Zucchinis

Filling:
Sweet soya sauce
Fresh coriander
Shelled walnuts

Sauce:
EVOO
Pepper
Vegetable broth

Bring water to boil in your rice cooker. Add EVOO & brown rice vermicelli or whole-grain angel hair pasta. Meanwhile, cut a thin slice lengthways along the top of each zucchini & chop finely. Using a teaspoon, scoop out the flesh from the middle of the zucchini & chop. Pre-heat oven to 400°. Place hollowed zucchini in an ovenproof dish and set aside.

To make filling: Place 2/3 cup of sweet soya sauce & garlic in wok. Add 3 TBSP of chopped fresh coriander, followed by 1/3 cup of shelled walnuts finely chopped. Stir in cooked vermicelli. Using a teaspoon, stuff each zucchini with the filling. Cover with aluminum foil and bake for 20 minutes.

Meanwhile make sauce: Place 4 TBSP EVOO, garlic, 1 cup of chopped fresh coriander, pepper, 3 TBSP of vegetable broth & pre-scooped out zucchini flesh in food processor or blender. Heat the sauce and pour over stuffed zucchini and serve. Garnish with finely chopped walnuts.

Really Supercharged Peppers

Pre-heat the oven to 350°. Oil an oven safe pan and set aside for later. Cook the whole-grain rice or barley according to the directions on the box.

Sautee some onions, sliced cherry tomatoes, artichoke hearts, fresh basil and parsley, lemon zest and juice

Remove and discard the tops of all the bell peppers. If the bell peppers are having trouble sitting up on their own, cut the bottoms of the peppers.

In a bowl, mix the rice/barley, tomatoes, and onion. Add the rice mixture to the hollowed bell peppers. (Optional) Prepare black beans to layer on top.

Bake 25-30 minutes

Really Simple Sweet Potatoes

Place sweet potatoes into baking dish. Slit each sweet potato with knife. Add about 1/4 inch of water to the baking dish. Cover with foil and bake at 350° for 45 minutes—1 hour. Add a pat of butter and spinkle with cinnamon.

Serve with sautéed spinach or any dark leafy green and herbs/ spices.

Really Soothing Soup

Cut the following vegetables into 1 inch pieces:carrots, potatoes, onions, yellow peppers & broccoli.

Saute in a large pot with 3 tablespoons of EVOO for a few minutes.

Stir in 2 cloves of fresh garlic & add low sodium organic tomato soup (in carton) & 2 cups of water. Cover & stir occasionally until done (approx 30 minutes).

In rice cooker: Add Barley & Quinoa to water and cook until done (approx 25 minutes).

Mix barley & quinoa with soup and add Himalayan salt, dried rosemary & garnish.

Serve with Cornbread

Cornbread Liquid Ingredients: 1½ cup of almond milk, 1½ TBSP Vinegar (ACV), 2 TBSP EVOO

Cornbread Dry Ingredients:1 cup cornmeal, 1 cup whole wheat flour, 2tsp coconut sugar, 1 tsp baking powder, ½ tsp baking soda
Mix the dry and liquid ingredients and bake at 425° for 20-25 min.

Anything Meals

Re-introduce E-Pizzas

Pre-heat oven to 350°. Place Ezekiel wraps on pan and add pizza/pasta sauce. Add your favorite toppings. Add fresh basil & dried herbs. Top with buffalo mozzarella cheese. Bake for 5-7 minutes and serve.

Re-explore Chicken Kabobs

Squash cut into one inch pieces
Zucchini cut into one inch pieces
Cherry tomatoes
Red pepper cut into one inch pieces
White onion cut into one inch pieces
Braggs Vinaigrette
Pineapple chunks

Directions:

Pre-heat oven to 350°. Place sliced squash, zucchini, and cherry tomatoes, red peppers and onions in a large bowl with vinaigrette. Let marinate in refrigerator until the chicken is ready. Season boneless skinless chicken breasts and bake in the oven for 30 minutes or until mostly done. Drain vegetables, reserving marinade. Place vegetables alternately with pineapple onto skewers. Place on pan and bake for 10-15 minutes, turning occasionally and basting with reserved marinade.

Serve alone or over whole-grain rice.

Re-infuse Turkey Burgers

Put the ground turkey into a mixing bowl and add the spices. Thyme, parsley, and sage are great spices to use. Also add minced onion, chopped fresh cilantro, Himalayan salt, and white pepper. (optional)hot peppers. Form patties and place on counter-top grill until done.

Serve with sweet potato fries, yucca fries, carrot fries or a salad.

Re-Create Spaghetti & Meatballs

Whole-grain Pasta
> Before you start the meatballs, use your rice cooker to cook your whole-grain spaghetti.

Turkey Meatballs

> Ingredients:
> 1 Package of ground turkey
> 1 large egg
> 1 small onion
> 1/4 cup of grated parm cheese
> 3 garlic cloves
> 1 oz of cold water
> Herbs (dried and/or fresh):pepper,thyme,oregano and basil
> 1/2 cup of dry bread crumbs (I toasted 2 pieces of whole-grain bread and crushed them)
>
> ~Mix everything together with hands and shape into balls and put in pan with EVOO and saute until brown. (Optional) Put in oven on 350° for 20-25 minutes.

Pasta Sauce
> Pour (preferably homemade) tomato pasta sauce over spaghetti. Garnish with parmesan cheese, green onions & cracked pepper.
>
> (Optional) You can sautee some chopped zucchini and add to sauce.

Re-form Shrimp Cakes

4 tablespoons extra virgin olive oil

1 teaspoon minced garlic

½ pound(8 ounces) shrimp peeled & deveined

4 cups cooked jasmine rice

2 teaspoons minced basil

2 teaspoons minced mint

2 teaspoons minced cilantro

2 teaspoons Siraccha

2 egg whites

1/4 cup finely sliced scallions for garnish

(Variation) Add dill weed and peas for a twist

Combine all ingredients except scallions in a medium-sized bowl. Using your hands, scoop enough of the mix to make 11/2-2 inch patties by squeezing and shaping, just as you would meatballs. Heat a large skillet over medium-high heat and add half of the oil.

Press the balls into the pan and cook for 4 minutes or until crispy and lightly browned. Flip with a spatula and brown the other side. Be sure to leave space in the pan between each patty so that they have enough heat to brown well.

Repeat until all of the patties are cooked. Serve immediately over a large bed of mixed greens.

Re-emerge Rainbow Taco Salad

Ingredients:

1 head of romaine lettuce, chopped

1 yellow onion

1/4 cup of chopped green onions

1/4 cup of chopped fresh cilantro

4 tomatoes diced

2 avocados cut in small pieces

1/2 cup chopped red peppers

1/2 cup chopped yellow peppers

1 cup black olives

1 carrot, medium shredded

2 tablespoons of lime juice

1 tsp ground Cumin

1/4 tsp pepper

7 ounces kidney beans drained and rinsed

7 ounces black beans drained and rinsed

1 cup of cheddar cheese

1/2 cup of organic salsa

1 bag of organic unsalted blue tortilla chips

DIRECTIONS:

(Remember to soak beans overnight)

Bring water to a boil in your rice cooker & then add EVOO and beans. **Make sure to use twice as much water to beans.** until tender.

Combine the onion, green onions, tomatoes, avocados, red and yellow peppers, black olives in a large bowl. In a separate small bowl mix the lime juice, cumin and pepper and then stir it into the larger bowl. Place the blue tortilla chips on the individual serving plates. Spoon the beans onto the blue tortilla chips. Spoon the vegetable mix from the large bowl onto the beans. Sprinkle with fresh cilantro. Top with romaine lettuce and cheddar cheese. Drizzle with salsa.

Serve immediately.

Re-experience Perfect Pancakes

Ingredients:

2 cups Arrowhead Mills Buttermilk Pancake & Waffle Mix

11/2 cups of water

Juice from half an orange

2 eggs

1 tsp. vanilla

11/2 tsp. baking powder butter

(Optional)1 tsp. lemon juice or lemon zest

(Optional) ¼ cup of whole pecans

Stir in all ingredients (except butter) until lumps disappear. Cook on preheated (350°-400°F) lightly buttered griddle or pan, turning when bubbles form on surface and edges begin to dry.

Serve immediately with Organic maple syrup.

Made in the USA
Coppell, TX
28 June 2022

79339911R10107